THE COMPLETE BOOK OF ESSENTIAL OILS FOR MAMA & BABY

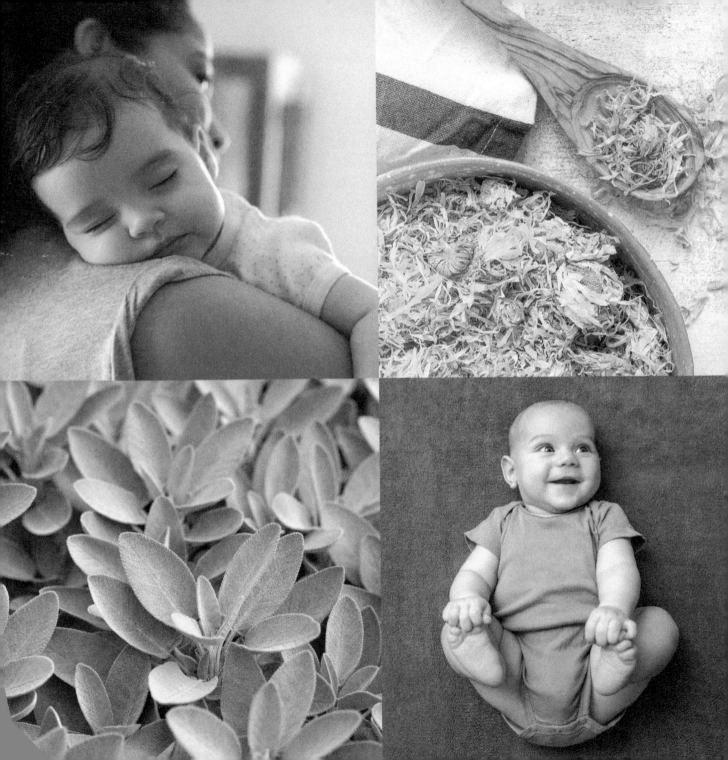

THE COMPLETE BOOK OF

Essential Oils

FOR Mama & Baby

Safe and Natural Remedies for Pregnancy, Birth, and Children

CHRISTINA ANTHIS

Foreword by Demetria Clark
Founder, Heart of Herbs Herbal School

ALTHEA
PRESS

For general information on our other products and services or to obtain technical support, please contact our Customer Care Department within the U.S. at (866) 744-2665, or outside the U.S. at (510) 253-0500.

Althea Press publishes its books in a variety of electronic and print formats. Some content that appears in print may not be available in electronic books, and vice versa.

TRADEMARKS: Althea Press and the Althea Press logo are trademarks or registered trademarks of Callisto Media Inc. and/or its affiliates, in the United States and other countries, and may not be used without written permission. All other trademarks are the property of their respective owners. Althea Press is not associated with any product or vendor mentioned in this book.

Photography © Marlon Lopez MMG1 Design/Shutterstock.com, cover; p. ii (clockwise from top right): Shannon Douglas; Andrii Orlov/Shutterstock.com; Pixeljoy/Shutterstock.com; Monkeybusinessimages/iStock; p. viii (clockwise from top right): Atle Rønningen/Stocksy; Mapodile/iStock; Claus Mikosch/Shutterstock.com; Borislav Zhuykov/Stocksy; p. 2 (clockwise from top right): Amy Covington/Stocksy; PeopleImages/iStock; Shannon Douglas; p. 10 (clockwise from top right): JRP Studio/Shutterstock.com; Courtney Rust/Stocksy; Sunny Forest/Shutterstock.com; p. 34 (clockwise from top right): Xpixel/Shutterstock.com; Raymond Forbes LLC/Stocksy; Elvira Koneva/Shutterstock.com; p. 80 (clockwise from top right) Janaph/Shutterstock.com; Christian B/Stocksy; Bernd Schwabedissen/iStock; p. 110 (clockwise from top right): Allen WorldWide/Shutterstock.com; Alija/iStock; Africa Studio/Shutterstock.com.

Illustrations © Kelsey Garrity-Riley 2017

ISBN: Print 978-1-62315-934-4 | eBook 978-1-62315-935-1

TO SILAS THOR,
YOU WILL ALWAYS BE
MY MIRACLE

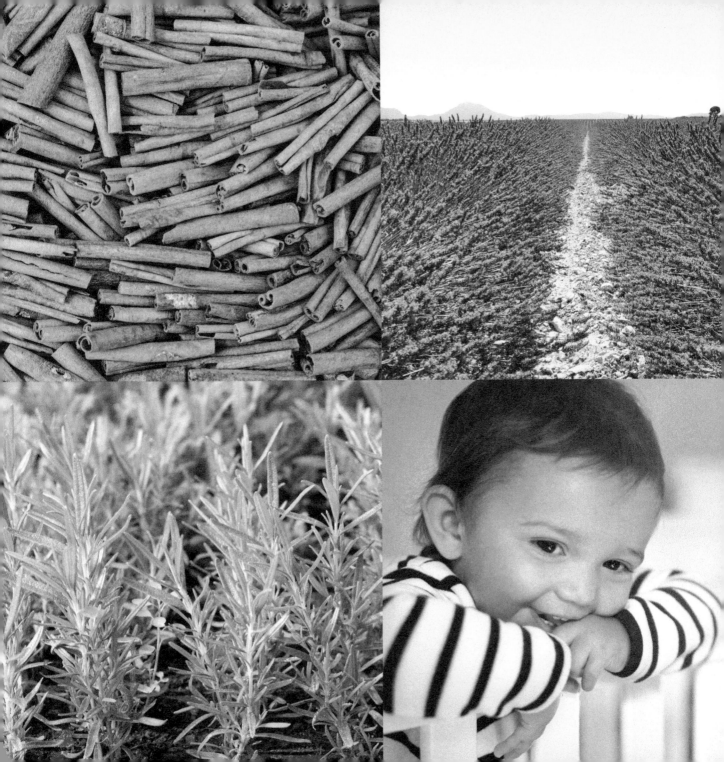

THE HEALING POWER
OF ESSENTIAL OILS

Pregnancy is a miracle, but it can also come with many aches and pains. After birth, we want to do everything we can to keep our little ones healthy. Essential oils can help you keep your family healthy without all of the worrisome side effects Western medicines may produce. Here are a few essential oils remedies for common pregnancy and postpartum issues.

MORNING SICKNESS

Despite the name, morning sickness can strike at any time of day. Inhaling essential oils of ginger, citrus, or spearmint can help calm nausea and soothe an upset stomach. See page 65 for helpful morning sickness remedies.

DRY/CRACKED NIPPLES

One of the most common discomforts that breastfeeding mothers experience is dry and/or cracked nipples. You can easily combat this issue by making a simple nipple cream using coconut oil and German chamomile essential oil. See page 101 for soothing salves.

DIAPER RASH

Diaper rash is the result of too much moisture on a baby's bum, causing irritation. Lavender essential oil has antibacterial properties and is a natural pain reliever, making it the perfect gentle addition for homemade Baby Butt Balm (page 164). See page 164 for other tried-and-true treatments.

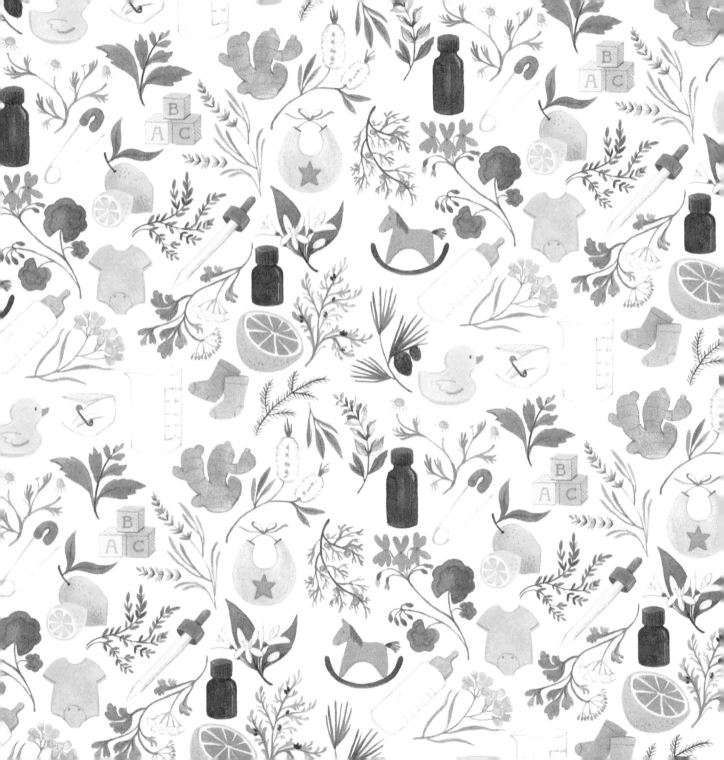

Contents

Foreword

I HAVE ALWAYS BEEN PASSIONATE ABOUT THE HEALING PROPERTIES OF PLANTS. Through my experience as the Director of the Heart of Herbs Herbal School, and as the author of several books on essential oils and aromatherapy, I've come to understand that parents crave safe, evidence-based information that gives them confidence and security when using natural remedies with their children.

At the same time, there are moments when you need a solution *right now*, like when your little one feels pain in the middle of the night and you're hesitant to reach for the bottle of over-the-counter medication, with its potentially harmful side effects. In those moments, *The Complete Book of Essential Oils for Mama and Baby* makes for an excellent resource. It fully expresses my personal motto—"keep it simple and useful"—by providing essential oils formulas that are simple to implement and, beyond that, actually work.

These days, essential oils are one of the most popular alternative healing modalities, but with that comes a lot of misinformation. Misinformation leads to unsafe practices that can make essential oil use scary for many. But with this book, you can trust that the essential oils remedies specify safe amounts for you and your little one.

If you're new to essential oils, this book lays it all out for you. I love so much of what Christina delivers, including informative profiles of "30 Family-Friendly Essential Oils to Know," which covers the most-used essential oils, and makes shopping for essential oils easy—easy being of the utmost importance when you're a busy mom. Christina has also included a comprehensive rating of various essential oils brands and very practical advice on shopping for your oils, which is a necessary step in the process of your essential oils education. Before you hand over your hard-earned dollars, you definitely want to understand what to look for and what to avoid when shopping. I know it can be difficult to avoid tempting claims on labels and sales pitches, so being an informed shopper makes all the difference in your overall experience and purchase power. In this book, Christina makes it simple for you to access high quality oils at affordable prices.

However, the most important aspect of this book is its spotlight on the safe use of essential oils, particularly when it comes to treating our children, the most sensitive of beings. Like all other healing methods, there are correct and incorrect ways to use essential oils. Christina expertly drills down into the practicalities of safe use, including information on which oils you can use freely for children of all ages, and which should be avoided, depending on your child's age.

As a former instructor, I know how overwhelming learning can be, and I am thrilled that with this delightful, practical book my former pupil has created such a wonderful resource for families that will benefit them for years to come.

DEMETRIA CLARK
founder, Heart of Herbs Herbal School;
author of *Herbal Healing for Children*
and *Aromatherapy and Herbal Remedies*
for Pregnancy, Birth, and Breastfeeding

Introduction

I THOUGHT THAT MOTHERHOOD WASN'T IN THE CARDS FOR ME. For years, I'd struggled with reproductive problems due to polycystic ovarian syndrome (PCOS), endometriosis, and a retroverted uterus. When I started to experience sudden waves of nausea, it never occurred to me that it might be morning sickness. My husband and I had not planned to get pregnant. So it would not be an understatement to say we were shocked—in the very best way—to learn I was pregnant and that we were going to be parents after all.

My pregnancy was not an easy one. Morning sickness did not go away after the first trimester, and I had trouble keeping anything but crackers down when nausea would hit. Desperate to find a safe solution, a close friend of mine suggested I try using aromatherapy to ease my symptoms. At first I thought she was a little nutty for thinking the smell of an oil could do anything to help, but I was willing to try just about anything. She suggested that I try inhaling ginger essential oil at the start of my nausea, so I bought my first bottle of essential oil and gave it a go the next time my nausea hit. I was amazed when it helped calm my nausea and soothe my stomach. I was able to eat an entire sandwich for lunch and it didn't come back up!

That day was the beginning of my essential oils obsession. I had to know more.

- What was the science behind their usage?

- Why did these oils work?

- What safety precautions did I need to know about?

- What other ailments could I use them for?

I spent hours reading books and scouring websites for information but found a lot of contradictory advice. Confused as to what was safe and what was not, I decided to take the plunge and start my studies for a clinical aromatherapy certification through Heart of Herbs online school, taught by Demetria Clark, a renowned herbalist, aromatherapist, and midwife.

It didn't take me long to realize that essential oils are wonderful, natural tools that can be used for many different purposes, and can produce amazing results—when used safely.

After studying the science and safe usage of essential oils, I noticed that a lot of the advice offered online, and surprisingly, even in many aromatherapy books, was unsafe.

Essential oil safety became my main passion and focus in my writing and on my blog. I created this book to be your ultimate guide to safe usage of essential oils throughout your pregnancy, delivery, postpartum, and even while raising your little humans. Whether you are pregnant and dealing with morning sickness, swollen ankles, and round ligament pains, or your little one has caught a cold with the sniffles and a cough, you will be able to find safe remedies for all your needs!

This book is laid out in an easy-to-read format so that you can quickly find the safe advice you are looking for in your time of need.

PART 1 covers general safety guidelines and use, the science of essential oils, what to look for in an essential oil brand, and handy reference charts that list which essential oils are safe to use through all stages of pregnancy and breastfeeding, as well as with babies and young children.

PART 2 is the heart of the book, and offers 200 essential oil blends and remedies, organized alphabetically by ailments and issues, for the prepartum and postpartum stages.

PART 3 helps you delve deeper into common individual essential oils and their uses and benefits. I've included profiles of 30 essential oils that are safe to use during pregnancy and breastfeeding, and noted those safe to both use around and to treat young children.

The book concludes with resources, including a glossary, an ailments and oils quick-reference guide, my favorite oils for labor kits, and a guide to picking the right essential oil brands for your family.

With this book, you will learn to incorporate essential oils safely and effectively throughout your entire motherhood journey, no matter what issues arise. When used properly, these oils can help you to keep your entire family healthy and happy, from pregnancy to birth and beyond!

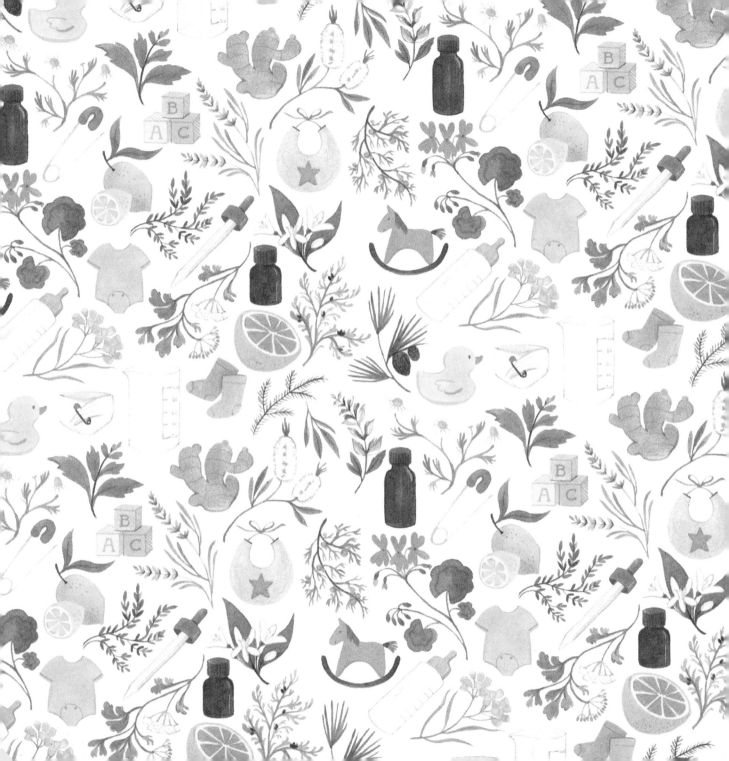

PART ONE

Safe & Natural Essential Oils

Whether you're a new mom or getting ready to add to your growing family, motherhood will throw you a few curveballs before, during, and after delivery.

In this chapter, you will be introduced to essential oils, their benefits and uses, the science behind how they work, and how to obtain the best quality essential oils. Safety is of the utmost concern, so in chapter 2 we'll explore all your safety concerns, including learning about carrier oils, methods of application, and how to modify essential oils used at every stage and age.

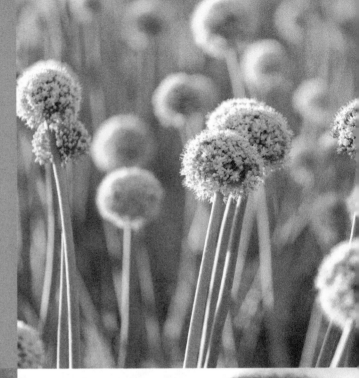

CHAPTER
ONE

The Natural Power of Essential Oils

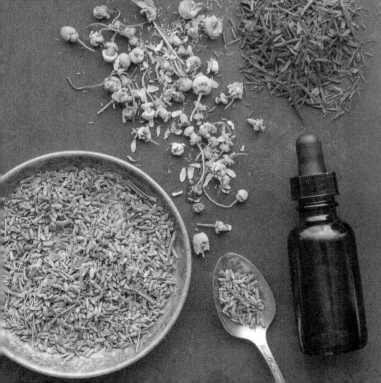

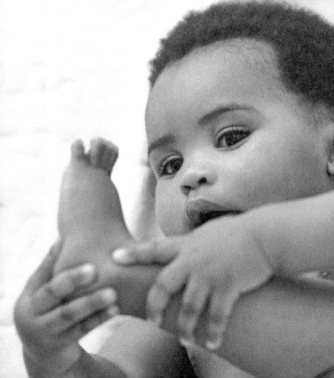

IT SEEMS EVERYONE IS TALKING ABOUT ESSENTIAL OILS these days—they've become the newest and hottest health trend. Would it surprise you to learn that essential oils have been used for centuries? The ancient Egyptians perfected the use of aromatic oils and herbs to create cosmetic and medicinal concoctions—many of which we use, albeit in different forms, today. Through trade, the knowledge of their medicinal uses carried over from culture to culture. But the birth of modern medicine went down a different path, society followed, and slowly we forgot the knowledge passed down for centuries.

It wasn't until an accident in 1910 that modern science began to take notice of the healing benefits of essential oils. When René-Maurice Gattefossé, a French perfume chemist, experienced a lab explosion, his hands, covered in chemical burns, soon developed a serious infection—gas gangrene. On a hunch, he applied lavender essential oil to the necrotic sores. To his delight, one application of lavender essential oil completely stopped the "gasification of the tissue." Following this discovery, he continued researching essential oils, using his knowledge to help treat soldiers in World War I. He eventually published his seminal 1937 book, *Aromathérapie*, also the first time the word "aromatherapy" was seen in print.

Yet it wasn't until after World War II when aromatherapy became widely recognized by Western physicians. Among others, the world owes much to Dr. Jean Valnet, a French physician. He'd studied Gattefossé's work, and as an army surgeon in World War II, used essential oils to help treat his own patients. From 1959 until his death in 1995, he dedicated his practice to herbal medicine and the medicinal use of essential oils, authoring many definitive works on the subject.

We've truly come full circle. Essential oils are in the spotlight for all the right reasons, yet people are simply relearning what so many already knew: Essential oils are more than just perfume. Essential oils are tools we can use to naturally enhance our health and our lives.

What Are Essential Oils?

Essential oils are highly concentrated aromatic oils extracted from flowers, leaves, grasses, fruits, roots, and trees. These oils contain the volatile compounds from the plants they are extracted from, many of which are isolated for use in pharmaceutical medicine. Used in everything from cosmetics and soap, to healing salves, and even cleaning supplies, essential oils are diverse in their uses and have many impressive healing qualities to them. The simple act of smelling certain essential oils can even lighten a mood or room, calm an anxious mind, or help you to focus when your mind wants to stray from the task at hand.

Depending on what part of the plant is being used, there are several methods to extract essential oils:

STEAM DISTILLATION   Most essential oils are made through steam distillation. During this method, plant material is loaded into a pot along with water and is sealed shut. The plant material is broken down by the steam and the essential oils rise up with the steam and flow through a tube into a condenser. The condenser cools the rising steam and essential oils back into liquid form and hydrosol and essential oils are produced. Since oil and water do not mix, the oil floats on top of the hydrosol and is siphoned off to separate the two.

COLD-PRESSED   This method of extraction is most often used for citrus, including lemon, bergamot, sweet orange, bitter orange, tangerine, blood orange, and grapefruit. Citrus essential oil is all in the peel! When you bite through the skin of an orange and feel the sting on your lips along with the slightly bitter taste of peel, this is your skin reacting to the undiluted citrus essential oil. Citrus peels can also be steam distilled, but the cheapest method of extraction is cold-pressing. The peels are chopped up and soaked in water before pressing the water and oils out. The oil is then siphoned off to separate the essential oil from the water and any juice.

ABSOLUTES AND CO$_2$ (CARBON DIOXIDE) EXTRACTS   When plant material is too fragile to withstand distillation, the best method to use is solvent extraction. The method is often used to create more affordable essential oils of delicate flowers. There are many solvents that can be used to create absolutes and extracts, including ethanol, methanol, and hexane. During pregnancy, it's a good idea to stay away from most absolutes and other solvent-extracted essential oils because you cannot be sure if there might be any solvent left behind (traces of hexane have been found in many absolutes on

The Aromatherapy-Essential Oils Connection

If you are new to aromatherapy, you are likely wondering just how smelling something, like lavender essential oil, can help you sleep at night. Your nose acts as the first part of the olfactory system (your sense of smell). Your lungs have a huge surface area intimately connected to your bloodstream, and when directly inhaled, the molecules from essential oils can enter straight into the blood. This makes essential oils great at treating bronchial issues like a cough or a chest infection.

Olfaction is one of the most primal senses in the human brain. Smell is a chemical reaction that happens when receptors in your brain interact with the chemical components of anything that you smell. As early as 1923, Italian physicians Giovanni Gatti and Renato Cayola concluded that odor can have a huge effect on the central nervous system; in their research, they noticed that certain essential oils produced an immediate effect on respiration, pulse, and blood pressure. Other studies have shown that smells can have instant psychological and physiological effects. They can even control who you are attracted to and who you would like to stay far away from.

the market). According to the National Institute for Occupational Safety and Health (NIOSH), exposure to certain types of solvents during pregnancy can cause miscarriage, stillbirth, preterm birth, or even birth defects.

The Benefits of Essential Oils

Before I began learning about essential oils, I had no idea they could successfully be used in so many ways. It wasn't until I started profiling specific essential oils for my studies that I learned how useful a single oil could be. For example, I was delighted to discover that lavender essential oil could easily help heal up a deep cut on my finger, relax my mind for a good night's rest, and relieve muscle pain in my neck, all without any unwanted side effects. As I expanded my essential oil collection and used them more in my life, I began to notice my family's health improving. My monthly sinus infections disappeared, I slept better, and we fell sick less often. If anyone did catch a cold, it lasted only a fraction of the time it normally did and it didn't take down the entire house. Here are some of the benefits of using essential oils:

HEALTH AND WELLNESS Essential oils have countless benefits for health, ranging from having antibacterial and antiseptic properties, to anti-inflammatory and calming properties.

They are used in natural cosmetics instead of hormone-disrupting fragrances and have the ability to cleanse germs from household surfaces, making them an excellent replacement for toxic cleaning products.

NATURAL ALTERNATIVE If you are trying to do away with toxic chemicals, essential oils have the power to replace many over-the-counter medications without their side effects. Essential oils can help soothe a headache, heal an ear infection without the unneeded use of antibiotics (most ear infections are viral and don't require antibiotics), or even help you gently drift off to sleep.

SELF-EMPOWERMENT The moment I realized I didn't have to visit the doctor for every cough, sore throat, and cold was the moment that I put my health into my own hands. Knowing that I have the ability to take care of everyday illnesses that may arise is extremely empowering. The more you learn how to use essential oils in your own life, the more you will feel empowered to keep your family and friends healthy and happy.

BUDGET-FRIENDLY With a growing family, one of your main concerns is likely to be cost. One of the best things about using essential oils to keep your family healthy is that it is far easier on your wallet than copays and prescription prices. Essential oils are highly concentrated, so it doesn't take too many drops to get the job done. One bottle of lavender

essential oil can be used for multiple issues, helping you minimize the need to buy separate remedies for every problem.

A CLEANER ENVIRONMENT It might surprise you to learn many of the cosmetics, bath, and beauty products sold at your local grocery or big-box store contain ingredients that are not only toxic to you but also to the environment. Making or buying cleaning supplies containing essential oils instead of manufactured fragrances also helps clean the air in your home. Spraying an air freshener in your environment may seem like a harmless act, but instead of cleaning the air, it causes further chemical pollution. A study by the Environmental Working Group of over 20 cleaning supplies that are used in schools revealed many of these products contained a large amount of toxic ingredients that are not even disclosed on the product's ingredients list. Some of the most toxic ingredients are bronchial irritants that cause serious allergic reactions, asthma, migraines, cancer, and more!

The Science of Essential Oils

If you're like me, you may have mistakenly thought that essential oils are only used by massage therapists, new-agey types, or simply to make everything smell better, but it turns out there is solid science behind aromatherapy.

While we have centuries of anecdotal evidence pointing to the effectiveness of plant medicine, it's only in the last century that we have begun studying essential oils more in depth.

Though we don't have as many studies on essential oils as we do the hundreds of pharmaceuticals being sold on the market, many studies have started to pop up in the last decade or two in response to increased interest in the use of essential oils. Several recent studies have shown that multiple essential oils are extremely antibacterial, with cinnamon and clove essential oils showing the highest amount of antibacterial properties, even against E. coli. Another study published in the *Asian Pacific Journal of Tropical Biomedicine* concluded that eucalyptus essential oil has antimicrobial activity against gram-negative bacteria (such as E. coli) as well as gram-positive bacteria. One of my favorite all-around essential oils, lavender, has a whole lot more than just antibacterial and antifungal properties. Lavender essential oil has been proven to be a powerful anti-inflammatory as well as an analgesic.

From basic chemistry we know that everything in life is made up of chemicals, and that includes essential oils. Each essential oil is made up of chemical constituents (or as I like to call them, ingredients). Every essential oil has a different makeup of these constituents, and many share several of the same ones, just in different amounts. Many constituents of essential oils are also isolated in industrial labs for use in medicine, pesticides, cleaning supplies, food flavoring, food preservation, and more.

The Best Essential Oil Brand

Everyone wants to know: Which is the *best* brand of essential oils? Many people will swear by just one or another, asserting its oils are the purest, the most unadulterated. On my quest to find the best essential oils, I was surprised to learn there is no governing body that certifies essential oils, and there are no grades for their quality either. Terms like "Certified Pure Therapeutic Grade™" or "Therapeutic Grade™" are misleading because they are actually trademarked marketing terms, rather than a classification of purity. I try to avoid those essential oil companies that market their essential oils by purity; instead, I look for a few key factors when I am buying essentials:

LABELING, INGREDIENTS, AND COUNTRY OF ORIGIN. A reputable essential oils company will label all its essential oils appropriately with the Latin name of the essential oil and the country of origin. The ingredients should solely be the essential oil, and should not also include a carrier oil unless you are intentionally buying a blend.

DO THEY PROMOTE THE UNSAFE USE OF ESSENTIAL OILS?   While aromatherapy is a wonderful natural modality that can be used in multiple ways, there are many companies in the United States that take advantage of insufficient regulation and promote unsafe use of essential oils for the sake of profits. I do not personally buy from companies that promote internal ingestion. *Ingesting essential oils is unsafe unless you are a healthcare practitioner trained at the appropriate clinical level.*

DO THEY SELL ESSENTIAL OILS OF PLANTS THAT ARE ENDANGERED?   There are countless companies that harvest and use essential oils of endangered plants. Always consider where your essential oil has come from and if it is extracted from an endangered plant species. You can keep track of current endangered aromatic species on CropWatch.unl.edu

ARE THEY AN ECO-CONSCIOUS COMPANY? I am passionate about the environment. How much a company that sells natural products cares about the natural world makes a huge difference in where I put my dollars.

So you can probably tell that I don't believe there is, without question, a single "best" brand of essential oils. Given the factors I consider, my favorites are Plant Therapy and Mountain Rose Herbs. Plant Therapy has a passion for kid-safe use, so much so that they created a kid-safe line of essential oil blends and singles. Every blend is created with essential oils that are safe for children 2 years and older. Mountain Rose Herbs is a certified zero-waste company that carries only certified organic herbs, essential oils, and other natural ingredients. You will find links to these and other brands in Appendix C (page 259).

What's Next?

In the next chapter, we'll take a closer look at the basics of essential oil safety during each stage of your pregnancy, labor, and delivery, as well as safe use for babies and growing children. You will also find more information about dilution and how to properly dilute essential oils for the next nine months and beyond.

Essential Oil Safety for Nine Months & Beyond

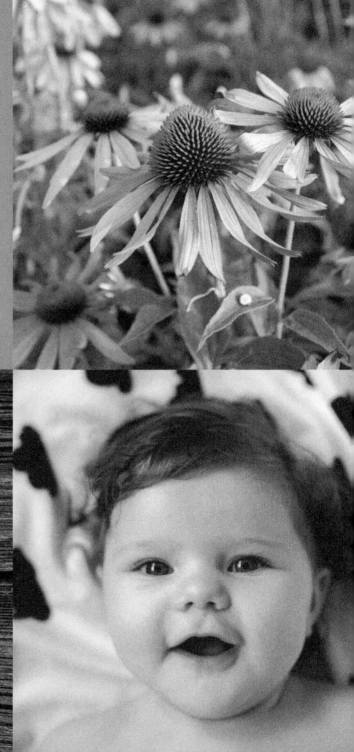

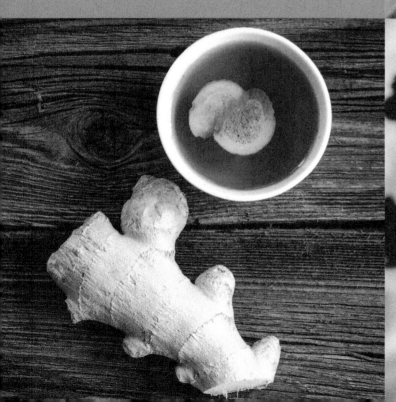

PREGNANCY, CHILDBIRTH, AND CHILDREN ARE MAGNIFICENT—
a time of magic and miracles—but each stage is not without its challenges.
Essential oils can help you through the tough times when you are sad
or anxious over the new responsibilities of being a mother, or even help
to soothe your little one and make them more comfortable when illness
strikes. I hold a special place in my heart for essential oils because I first
discovered them during my pregnancy with my son, Silas. I was bedridden
and nauseated most of the time, but with the help of ginger and sweet
orange essential oil, I managed to keep my food down and a smile on my
face. After Silas was born, I used lavender and lemon essential oils to heal
my C-section scar, and fir needle essential oil to soothe my baby's cough
and congestion. Essential oils were an excellent resource for me from the
beginning of my journey into motherhood, and continue to be so, now,
helping me keep my family happy and healthy.

Safety First

When it comes to children and their mothers, nothing is more important than safety. Educating others on the safe use of essential oils, especially as they pertain to babies and small children, has become my life's work.

With the rising costs of healthcare and numerous side effects from pharmaceuticals use, we are fortunate to have these natural remedies and preventative approaches at our fingertips. These precious plant essences are an affordable option that anyone can use. This chapter covers everything you must know before getting started with the recipes to make your own essential oil remedies in the next part. It is important that you familiarize yourself with the basic rules for essential oil safety before getting started.

The Importance of Dilution

It takes quite a bit of plant matter to fill that little bottle with precious drops of essential oils. The oils are highly concentrated and dilution with a carrier oil (a "neutral" oil, which we'll discuss in the next section) is key to safe usage. When using essential oils to treat pregnant women, babies, and small children, the essential oil should *always* be diluted. If undiluted and applied directly to the skin, essential oils can cause irritation and burning, or worse yet, sensitization. Sensitization occurs when your body develops an allergy to an essential oil or one of the constituents in it. Marge Clarke, in her introductory aromatherapy book *Essential Oils and Aromatics*, put her personal experience with sensitization very powerfully: "Years ago, I read the books saying that lavender oil could be used neat (undiluted). I unwisely used undiluted lavender on broken skin, and consequently set up a sensitivity reaction. Today, almost two decades later, if I come in contact with lavender in any form, I will immediately experience dermatitis that can take months to heal."

HYDROSOLS & BEAUTY CLAYS

Hydrosols are made from the condensed vapor from the processing of essential oils. More gentle than neat (undiluted) essential oils, they can be safely used on newborns, and most can be used in place of water in any recipe. They are available from most essential oil manufacturers. All of the companies mentioned in Appendix C (page 259), except for Aura Cacia and NOW Foods, sell hydrosols.

CARRIER OILS

Often referred to as base oils or fixed oils, carrier oils are not the same as essential oils. While essential oils are volatile (they evaporate) and extremely concentrated, carrier oils are base vegetable oils (many of which are in your own pantry already) that are cold-pressed and used to dilute and "carry" essential oils. They are often used in cosmetics for their moisturizing and healing properties, and in massage oils for their natural glide. Any lotion, butter, or soap you own contains some form of carrier oil in its ingredients list. While there are many types of carrier oils, these are my five favorites to keep on hand for all my aromatherapy needs:

1. AVOCADO SEED OIL   We all know avocados are good for you, but their awesome benefits don't stop at eating them. Easy to find at the grocery store, refined avocado oil has little to no smell, is clear in color, and is deeply moisturizing to dry skin and hair. I love to use avocado oil in my facial moisturizing oil, to deeply condition my hair, and in my whipped body butters. Avocado oil is heavier than most, making it great for moisturizing applications.

2. COCONUT OIL/FRACTIONATED COCONUT OIL   One of my favorite oils! In its unrefined state, it hardens in temperatures colder than 76°F, making it a favorite choice of

Feeling Scent-sitive?

One of the most interesting superpowers of pregnancy is the intensity with which you can smell the world. During my pregnancy I had such an aversion to the smell of garlic that I had to avoid all foods that had garlic cooked in them, and even the kitchen at times. Being aromatic by nature, certain essential oils can cause scent aversion for some pregnant women. This is different for every woman, so the best option is to first take a brief whiff from the essential oil bottle to be sure that your nose gets along with that scent. Certain overpowering essential oils, including geranium and ylang-ylang, may need to be heavily diluted because their scents can be overpowering even if you aren't pregnant. If you find yourself with a scent aversion, try sniffing sweet orange essential oils to "cleanse" your nose's palate.

mine for simple salves. Naturally antibacterial, antifungal, antiseptic, and anti-inflammatory, coconut oil is healing and soothing to the skin and can even be applied to cuts and scrapes with lavender essential oil as a simple antibacterial cream for small cuts and scrapes. Fractionated coconut oil does not harden like unrefined coconut oil and has no smell, making it a great carrier oil to use in essential oil roll-on applications. Because coconut oil is actually fairly *comedogenic* (that means it can clog your pores), I would suggest avoiding it in facial oils and moisturizers, but it's fantastic for all other applications.

3. GRAPESEED OIL Grapeseed oil is rich in the same antioxidants found in wine. This naturally anti-inflammatory oil has little scent, and it is one of the best oils for carrying aromatics for long periods of time, making it great for perfume-type blends and aromatherapy roll-ons. I frequently use this oil in my facial cleansing oil, salves, and even in scar cream. The oil sinks into skin pretty quickly and is non-comedogenic.

4. HEMP SEED OIL One of the best carrier oils to combat acne, hemp seed oil is rated the lowest on the comedogenic scale—it's the oil least likely to clog your pores. Hemp seed oil is wonderful in facial moisturizers, body butters, and lotions, because it absorbs quickly and leaves skin feeling extremely soft. Hemp seed oil has a defined nutty scent that can overpower the scent of some essential oils; you can diffuse the scent some if you mix it with another carrier oil.

5. OLIVE OIL If your house is anything like mine, olive oil is a staple carrier oil already in your kitchen. Guess what: It's great for so much more than sautéing onions and dressing salads. Rich in antioxidants and healing and nourishing to the skin, olive oil is great for many applications. Growing up, we used olive oil to moisturize our faces, condition our hair, and even fix a squeaky door. These days, I love to use this oil in all my healing salves. Naturally antibacterial, it mixes well with coconut oil to make herbal-infused oils for skin-healing salves and lip balms. Extremely moisturizing but a bit greasy, it works well by itself but even better when mixed with another carrier oil. Olive oil's strong scent can take over a blend if not mixed with another carrier oil.

NOTE: If you or your children have nut allergies, avoid using nut oils and coconut oil to prevent an allergic reaction. All of the other oils suggested above are nut allergy-friendly!

Five Herbs That Support a Healthy Pregnancy

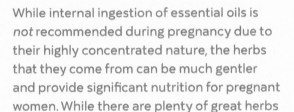

While internal ingestion of essential oils is *not* recommended during pregnancy due to their highly concentrated nature, the herbs that they come from can be much gentler and provide significant nutrition for pregnant women. While there are plenty of great herbs to choose from, these are my top five:

1. **RASPBERRY LEAF** Rich in vitamins C, E, B-complex, calcium, iron, phosphorus, potassium, niacin, magnesium, and manganese, raspberry leaf is used extensively by midwives around the world to strengthen, tone, and prepare the uterus for delivery. Raspberry leaf can easily be used in a tea, daily. You can begin drinking raspberry leaf tea every day, starting in the third trimester. To prepare, pour 8 to 10 ounces of freshly boiled water over 1 tablespoon of raspberry leaf. Cover the cup and steep for 10 to 15 minutes. To make this over ice, steep the tea for 30 minutes and pour over ice. You can enjoy 3 to 4 cups tea per day.

2. **NETTLE** Stinging nettle is a highly nutritious plant, rich in vitamins and minerals, including vitamins A, C, E, and K, as well as B vitamins, and silica. It is one of my favorite herbs to put in vitamin-rich teas because of its high vitamin and mineral content, and it's safe for consumption while pregnant. Nettle is also a diuretic herb; when combined with raspberry leaf it can safely heal up and prevent urinary tract infections, a common problem in pregnancy. It's becoming more common to see pre-packaged nettle teas in mainstream grocery stores, but if yours doesn't carry loose nettle, it can usually be found at natural food markets, herbal shops, or easily ordered online from Mountain Rose Herbs. (See Appendix C, page 259.)

3. **GINGER** A multifaceted and spicy culinary herb capable of some pretty amazing things, ginger is the hero to any pregnant woman experiencing morning sickness. When nausea strikes, either make a tea using fresh slices of ginger in boiling water, or chew on candied pieces of ginger.

4. **CHAMOMILE** Smelling of sweet apples, gentle chamomile is a favorite among herbalists. This digestive herb is great at soothing an upset stomach, gas, and even frazzled nerves. Drink a cup of this right before bedtime to get a better night's rest. However, chamomile is a member of the ragweed family and should be avoided if you have allergies.

5. **ALFALFA** Yet another super-nutritious herb, alfalfa is rich in vitamins and minerals including A, the full family of B vitamins, D, E, K, plus biotin, calcium, folic acid, iron, magnesium, and potassium. When you have a hospital birth, one of the first shots given to newborn babies is vitamin K, to prevent a rare disease that causes brain hemorrhaging. If you are planning on having a natural birth at home, you can still supplement vitamin K by taking alfalfa supplements daily during the third trimester of your pregnancy. Alfalfa is also delicious blended in tea.

Recommended Dilution Amounts

All of the blends presented in chapter 3 of this book take into account proper dilution amounts. When you're ready to start experimenting on your own with essential oils (EO) and blends, here are the dilution amounts to follow:

Stage/Age	Max % EO Dilution	Max # of Drops per 1 oz Carrier
pregnancy	1%	9 drops
breastfeeding	2%	18 drops
babies 3–6 mo.	0.1%	1 drop
babies 6 mo.–2 yr.	0.5%	4–5 drops
children 2–6 yr.	1%	9 drops
children 6+ yr.	1.5%–2%	13–18 drops

Application Methods

Essential oils work in many ways to help the body, but there are three main ways that they are used:

TOPICAL Topical applications go directly on the skin. These applications are commonly used to treat the skin itself, using salves and creams to heal cuts, scrapes, burns, eczema, acne, and more. They can also be used for acute problems, including cough and congestion, muscle pain, and even menstrual pain. While topical application is great for skin conditions or acute issues, it is the slowest way to get essential oils into your bloodstream. A more heavily diluted oil blend will also take longer to get into the bloodstream.

AROMATIC Aromatic applications are inhaled. The fastest method of getting essential oils into the bloodstream, inhalation is one of the most effective and popular ways to use essential oils. Made up of a combination of chemical constituents, when inhaled these constituents travel to either your brain, your lungs, or both. Inhalation is actually one of the oldest methods of administering medications, and has recently been rediscovered in the mainstream pharmaceutical industry, with insulin and other therapies being administered through olfaction. Inhalation is also commonly used for respiratory tract infections, allergies, headaches, asthma, prevention of illness, depression, fatigue, nausea, insomnia, nicotine withdrawal, attention deficit/hyperactivity disorder (ADHD), and even stress and anxiety.

INGESTED Ingested applications go directly into the mouth. This method should *only* be performed under the guidance of a qualified medical professional. While there's a precedent for ingesting essential oils, *none of the remedies in this book should be ingested.*

Pregnancy

While essential oils can help alleviate many common pregnancy symptoms, it is especially important that you practice safe essential oil use to avoid any adverse reactions to you or your baby.

FIRST TRIMESTER

Aromatherapists agree that most essential oils should be avoided during the first three months of pregnancy, especially if you are high risk for a miscarriage. If you are experiencing morning sickness, peppermint or fresh ginger tea are effective herbal alternatives that can help alleviate those first symptoms of pregnancy.

SECOND AND THIRD TRIMESTER

After the first trimester has passed, it is safe to use essential oils sparingly throughout your pregnancy. During the second and third trimesters, use the following safety guidelines:

- Less is more with pregnant (and nursing) mamas! Always dilute essential oils with a carrier oil before use. You should not exceed

In the Event of a Miscarriage

The sudden loss of a child is devastating. While some aromatherapists might suggest an essential oil to massage onto your abdomen to stop a miscarriage, this can be unsafe without knowing the cause of the miscarriage. If you experience unexpected contractions, or heavy bleeding, consult with your midwife or medical practitioner immediately.

After a miscarriage, you may experience pain in your abdomen while your body is passing the remaining tissue. You might find some physical relief with a soothing massage of lavender and fir needle essential oils, diluted in a carrier. You may also apply clary sage to your lower abdomen, to help promote uterine contractions during this process as well. You can take a hot shower for cramping and pain, but avoid submerging your lower half in a bath or pool until the bleeding has stopped.

During this difficult time, it is important to communicate your feelings with your partner, family, or support team, and to work through this tough period together. Essential oils can be used in a diffuser to help ease the grief you may experience. Combine 7 drops grapefruit essential oil, 3 drops lavender essential oil, and 2 drops clary sage essential oil in your diffuser and diffuse throughout the room to help calm stress, relieve anxiety, and brighten the mood.

a 1 percent dilution, or 9 drops essential oil per 1 ounce of carrier oil.

- The diffuser should only run for 10 to 15 minutes at a time. Pregnant moms have sensitive noses and are susceptible to essential oil overexposure. Running the diffuser too long can cause headaches, nausea, and even dizziness. Take breaks!

- Minimize daily use as much as possible. It is best to utilize essential oils only when you need them, like helping with acute issues like nausea, indigestion, leg cramps and spasms, insomnia, cough and congestion, stress and anxiety, and more.

Labor & Delivery

The big day has arrived and you are about to meet the littlest member of your family! Essential oils can effectively help you through this laborious process. For best results, follow these safety guidelines when using essential oils during labor and in the delivery room.

LABOR

No two women's labor is the same. Some women experience long labor periods with little pain, while others will experience a ton of pain in a short amount of time, and everything in between is also possible. Essential oils can help you through the discomforts of labor if you follow these safety guidelines:

- Always dilute essential oils with a carrier oil before using. Don't exceed a 2 percent dilution, or 18 drops essential oil per 1 ounce of carrier oil.

- Run the diffuser for up to 30 minutes at a time. To avoid overexposure, it is best to set the diffuser to 30 minutes on/30 minutes off. Running the diffuser too long can cause headaches, nausea, and even dizziness.

DELIVERY

Just like labor, no two deliveries are the same. When using essential oils in the delivery room, it's important to follow these safety guidelines:

- Always dilute essential oils with a carrier oil. Don't exceed a 2 percent dilution, or 18 drops essential oil per 1 ounce of carrier oil.

- If using a birthing pool, *do not add essential oils to the pool.* Essential oils do not mix into water. Instead, they float on top. Adding essential oils to the birthing pool is dangerous to the newborn and could cause burns, irritation, and other problems.

48 HOURS AFTER DELIVERY

Those first two days of motherhood are going to fly by in a blur, and before you know it, you'll be bringing your beautiful bundle of joy home.

These safety guidelines will help you through the first 48 hours after birth:

- Always dilute essential oils with a carrier oil. Do not exceed a 2 percent dilution, or 18 drops essential oil per 1 ounce of carrier oil.

- Diffuse essential oils when your newborn is out of the room. Newborn babies are not ready to breathe essential oils just after birth.

- Avoid essential oil diffusion or use around premature babies. Babies born before 36 weeks are still developing their lungs and should not be around essential oils until they reach their 40 week due date.

- Do not apply essential oils to a C-section scar until the staples are removed or your doctor says you can.

Breastfeeding

If you choose to breastfeed your baby, there are a few safety guidelines to follow when using essential oils.

- Less is more. Breastfeeding mothers should not exceed a 2 percent dilution, or 18 drops essential oil per 1 ounce of carrier oil.

- Don't run the diffuser for more than 30 minutes at a time. To avoid essential oil overexposure, set the diffuser to a schedule of 30 minutes on/30 minutes off. Running it too long can lead to headaches, nausea, and dizziness.

- Apply nipple cream right after feeding, not before. This minimizes essential oil residue on the breast and accidental ingestion by your baby.

Babies

No matter their age, babies should never ingest essential oils orally. Keep all essential oils out of reach of babies and children. Certain essential oils may be toxic if ingested. Depending on the age of your baby, follow these safety guidelines to prevent any adverse reactions.

0 TO 3 MONTHS

Experts advise against the use of essential oils topically on babies less than 3 months of age because their immature skin is permeable and sensitive to essential oils. Unlike healthy adults, newborns' bodies are not capable of neutralizing adverse reactions to essential oils. Use even more caution with premature babies, avoiding essential oil use until they get 3 months past their due date. Only use diffusion for acute issues including nasal congestion or a cough. In other cases, hydrosols are a gentler option for newborns, when diffusion will not work. Avoid repeated daily use.

Five Herbs That Promote Lactation

Breastfeeding is such an amazing, natural, and cheap way to feed your baby everything they need to thrive, but as magical as this time can be for some breastfeeding mothers, it can be a whole different story for others. Consult with your lactation specialist or pediatrician if you think your baby is not getting enough nutrition or gaining enough weight. If you are having trouble producing milk, there are herbs that you can use to increase your milk production. My top five favorite herbs to promote lactation are:

1. **BLESSED THISTLE** A plant that has been a part of herbal medicine since before the Middle Ages, blessed thistle is a well known *galactogogue*, helping to stimulate the production of breast milk. It works extremely well when combined with fenugreek, fennel, or goat's rue. The most common ways to use blessed thistle while breastfeeding are in tea or capsule form. Prepare the tea by pouring 8 to 10 ounces of freshly boiled water over 1 to 2 teaspoons of loose blessed thistle. Cover the cup and steep the tea for 10 to 15 minutes before straining. You can enjoy up to 3 cups of this tea per day. When taking blessed thistle capsules, you can take up to 3 capsules 3 times per day. **Warnings:** You should avoid taking blessed thistle if you have an ulcer or other gastric issues. As a member of the ragweed family, it should be avoided if you are allergic to ragweed, daisies, and sunflowers. Blessed thistle should not be taken during pregnancy.

2. **FENUGREEK** A plant native to India, fenugreek has been used for centuries in cooking, flavoring, and medicine. It's especially great for digestive issues, but also has a long history associated with women's health including labor and delivery. Fenugreek is most effective when used to help promote lactation and is even used by dairy farmers to help increase the cow's milk supply. The most common ways to use fenugreek while breastfeeding are in tea or capsule form. Prepare the tea by pouring 8 to 10 ounces of freshly boiled water over 1 to 2 teaspoons of loose fenugreek seeds. Cover the cup and steep the tea for 10 to 15 minutes before straining. You can enjoy up to 3 cups of this tea per day. When taking fenugreek capsules, you can take 1 capsule 3 times per day. **Warnings:** This herb should be avoided during pregnancy because it can induce labor and cause a miscarriage. You should avoid using fenugreek if you are diabetic or hypoglycemic because it can lower blood sugar levels. Fenugreek can thin the blood, so it should be avoided if you are taking blood thinners.

3. **FENNEL** Commonly used in cooking, fennel is a wonderful healing herb that is also a powerful galactogogue and can help increase breast milk supply with its estrogen-like properties. Fennel has long

been used for digestive issues and can pass through the breast milk to help soothe a colicy baby as well. It is most commonly suggested to add fennel to your diet by eating it as a vegetable, drinking fennel tea, or using it to spice up your food. Prepare the tea by pouring 8 to 10 ounces of freshly boiled water over 1 to 2 teaspoons of freshly crushed fennel seeds. Cover the cup and steep the tea for 10 to 15 minutes before straining. You can enjoy up to 3 cups of this tea per day. **Warnings:** Fennel should be avoided during pregnancy. Fennel can increase the risk of a seizure and should be avoided if you have epilepsy, are prone to seizures, or take medication for seizures. You should avoid using fennel if you are diabetic or hypoglycemic because it can lower blood sugar levels.

4. GOAT'S RUE Native to Europe and the Middle East, goat's rue has been used for centuries in herbal medicine to increase breast milk production. A popular galactogogue, in Europe the dried leaves were even used to boost the milk supply in goats and cows. The most common ways to use goat's rue while breastfeeding are in tea or capsule form. Prepare the tea by pouring 8 to 10 ounces of freshly boiled water over 1 to 2 teaspoons of dried goat's rue leaves. Cover the cup and steep the tea for 10 to 15 minutes before straining. You can enjoy up to 3 cups of this tea per

day. When taking goat's rue capsules, you can take 1 capsule 3 times per day. **Warnings:** Goat's rue should only be used in its dried form. In its fresh form it is poisonous and should be avoided. You should avoid using goat's rue if you are diabetic or hypoglycemic because it can lower blood sugar levels. As a member of the pea family, it should be avoided if you are allergic to peanuts, soybeans, or alfalfa.

5. OATS A wonderful nutritive herb, all parts of the plant can be used to help support adequate mineral intake for lactating mothers to make more milk. Rich in magnesium, phosphorus, chromium, iron, calcium, B vitamins, and vitamins A and C, oats help to feed the nervous system and soothe frazzled nerves. According to the Herbal Academy of New England, oats are helpful during times of stress or exhaustion and can help to "mellow the mood, ease anxiety, combat the effects of daily stress, and resolve sleeplessness." Oats are commonly used in cold infusions, cooking, and baking, and can be prepared as oatmeal or added to smoothies and baked goods. To prepare a cold infusion, combine 1 cup oats (preferably dried oat tops, but any form of oats will work) with 1 quart of room temperature filtered water, and let steep overnight. Strain then store in the fridge and sip throughout the day.

Phototoxic Essential Oils

Certain citrus essential oils are phototoxic, meaning they may cause a red rash or sunburn around the spot where you apply an oil to your skin if you expose your body to the sun's rays, or UV lights, soon after application. Even a very small amount of some citrus oils can generate this reaction, while others you can safely use in small doses. Below I list the citrus oils that are phototoxic and should be used in moderation, as well as those that are safe.

PHOTOTOXIC OIL	MAX PER 1 OZ CARRIER OIL
Bergamot	4 drops
Bitter orange, cold-pressed	12 drops
Grapefruit	36 drops
Lemon, cold-pressed	18 drops
Lime, cold-pressed	6 drops
Mandarin leaf	2 drops

NON-PHOTOTOXIC

Bergamot (FCF or bergapten-free)	Mandarin
Lemon, steam-distilled	Orange leaf
Lemon leaf	Sweet orange
Lime, steam-distilled	Tangelo
	Tangerine

3 TO 6 MONTHS

At this age you can begin introducing your baby to essential oils, one at a time. It's important to introduce essential oils one at a time, in very small doses, then closely watch your baby for any sort of reaction or allergies, and allow your baby's body to slowly become accustomed to that essential oil. Do not introduce more than one essential oil in one day. Allow 24 hours to pass before introducing a new oil. A highly allergic reaction will occur in the first 15 to 30 minutes after inhalation or dermal application and can result in anaphylaxis. A minor reaction will occur within 24 hours after inhalation or dermal application and can result in dermal reaction. I recommend a 0.1 percent dilution, or 1 drop essential oil per 1 ounce of carrier oil for topical applications.

6 TO 24 MONTHS

As with babies aged 3 to 6 months, you should still be introducing new essential oils one at a time, to be sure that your baby does not have an allergy to any oils. I recommend a .0.5 percent dilution, or 4 to 5 drops essential oil per 1 ounce of carrier oil for topical applications.

2 TO 6 YEARS

At this age, children develop their physical motor skills and will get into plenty of scrapes for you to kiss and make better. As their sense of smell develops, you can involve them in choosing which essential oils they'd like in their blend. There are many different essential oils that can do the same job, so allowing your child to pick from two or three essential oils helps them learn more about which essential oils appeal to them and makes their blend more appealing because they made it themselves. I recommend a 1 percent dilution, or 9 drops essential oil per 1 ounce of carrier oil for topical applications.

NOTE: Children Should Never Ingest Essential Oils. Essential oils should never be given orally to children. According to Robert Tisserand in his book, *Essential Oil Safety*, "Most cases of essential oil poisoning involve accidents with young children, often between 1 and 3 years of age. Approximately 75 percent of cases in the USA are in children up to 6 years old."

If your child accidentally ingests essential oils, do not induce vomiting. Poison control advises to call your pediatrician unless signs of poisoning are present; then you should immediately bring your child and the container of the consumed essential oil to the nearest emergency room. Signs of poisoning can include diarrhea, stomach pain, drowsiness, dizziness, fever, loss of appetite, and headaches.

Nearly all essential oils are safe to use at this age. You can now teach your child how to safely apply their essential oil blends to themselves. Teach them to use a roll-on bottle or an aromatherapy inhaler so that they can carry your creations with them in their bags when they leave the house. I recommend a 1.5 to 2 percent dilution, or 13 to 18 drops per 1 ounce of carrier oil for topical applications.

Unsafe & Safe Oils

Whew! That was a lot of information in this relatively short chapter. If you're already experiencing "pregnancy brain"—little moments of forgetfulness here and there—you know there's no point in trying to remember every recommendation for every stage. This book is your reference, so simply refer to it when you need.

With that in mind, I've tried to make it incredibly easy to know which specific oils are not okay for you to use, and which are. The next several pages offer at-a-glance lists that you can turn to again and again. You might even want to snap a photo on your smartphone so you have access to them if you buy your oils in a store rather than online.

Essential Oils to Avoid

The following essential oils are toxic and should be avoided by everyone—pregnant or not.

Almond oil, bitter
Prunus dulcis

Boldo oil *Peumus boldus*

Cade oil *Juniperus oxycedrus*

Horseradish oil
Armoracia rusticana

Mustard oil *Brassica nigra*

Pine oil *Dacrydium franklinii*

Sassafras oil
Sassafras albidum

Sassafras oil, Brazilian
Nectandra sanguinea,
Ocotea odorifera

Sassafras oil, Chinese
Cinnamomum porrectum,
Cinnamomum rigidissimum

Snakeroot oil
Asarum canadense

Tea tree oil, black
Melaleuca bracteata

Wormseed oil
Henopodium ambrosioides

Essential Oils to Avoid While Pregnant or Nursing

The following essential oils should be avoided during pregnancy or while nursing because they may be abortifacient, cause harm to the fetus in some way, and can pass through the milk of a breastfeeding mother.

Aniseed *Pimpinella anisum*

Anise, Star *Illicium verum*

Araucaria *Neocallitropsis pancheri*

Artemisia *Artemisia vestita*

Atractylis *Atractylylodes lancea*

Lemon Basil *Ocimum x citriodorum*

Birch *Betula lenta*

Black Seed *Nigella sativa*

Buchu *Agathosma betulina, Agathosma crenulata*

Calamint *Calamintha nepeta*

Camphor *Cinnamomum camphora*

Carrot Seed *Daucus carota*

Cassia *Cinnamomum cassia*

Chaste Tree *Vitex ugnus castus*

Cinnamon Bark *Cinnamomum verum*

Essential Oils to Avoid While Pregnant or Nursing continued

Cypress, blue *Callitris intratopica*

Dill Seed *Anethum graveolens*

Dill Seed, Indian *Anethus sowa*

Eucalyptus *Eucalyptus camaldulensis, Eucalyptus globulus, Eucalyptus maidenii, Eucalyptus plenissima, Eucalyptus kochii, Eucalyptus polybractea, Eucalyptus radiata, Eucalyptus autraliana, Eucalyptus phellandra, Eucalyptus smithi*

Fennel, bitter and sweet *Foeniculum vulgare*

Feverfew *Tanacetum parthenium*

Frankincense *Boswellia papyrifer*

Genipi *Artemisia genepi*

Hibawood *Thujopsis dolobratta*

Ho Leaf *Cinnamomum camphora*

Hyssop *Hyssopus officinalis*

Lanyuna *Artemisia afra*

Lavender, French/Spanish *Lavandula stoechas*

Lemon Balm, Australian *Eucalyptus staigeriana*

Lemongrass *Cymbopogon flexuosus*

May Chang *Litsea cubeba*

Mugwort *Artemisia arborescens, Artemisia vulgaris*

Myrrh *Commiphora myrrha*

Myrtle, Honey *Melaleuca teretifolia*

Myrtle, Lemon *Backhousia citriodora*

Nutmeg *Mysristica fragrans*

Oregano *Origanum onites, Origanum smyrnaeum, Origanum vulgare, etc.*

Parsley, Leaf/Seed *Petroslinum sativum*

Pennyroyal *Mentha pulegium*

Peppermint *Mentha piperita*

Plectranthus *Plectranthus fruticosus*

Rosemary *Rosmarinus officinalis*

Rue *Ruta graveolens*

Sage, Dalmatian *Salvia officinalis*

Sage, Spanish *Salvia lavandulaefolia*

Tansy *Tanacetum vulgare*

Tea Tree, Lemon *Leptospermum petersonii*

Thuja *Thuja occidentalis*

Thyme, Lemon *Thymus x citriodorus*

Verbena, Lemon *Aloysia triphylla*

Western Red Cedar *Thuja plicata*

Wintergreen *Gaultheria procumbens*

Wormwood *Artemisia absinthium*

Yarrow *Achillea millefolium, Achillea nobilis*

Zeodary *Curcuma sedoaria*

Essential Oils Safe for Use While Pregnant or Nursing

The following essential oils have been proven safe to use in moderation while pregnant or nursing.

Clary Sage is marked with an asterisk (*) because it is not safe during pregnancy but may be used while nursing.

All of the oils listed are also generally considered safe to use around babies and young children.

Balsam Fir *Abies balsamea*

Bergamot *Citrus bergamia*

Black Pepper *Piper nigrum*

Blue Tansy *Tanacetum annuum*

Cedarwood, Virginia/Atlantic/Himalayan *Cedrus atlantica, Cedrus deodara, Juniperus virginiana*

Chamomile, German/Roman *Chamaemelum nobile, Matricaria recutita*

Citronella *Cymbopogon winterianus*

Clary Sage* *Salvia sclarea*

Copaiba *Copaifera langsdorfii, Copaifera officinalis*

Coriander *Coriandrum sativum*

Cypress *Cupressus sempervirens*

Dill Weed *Anethum graveolens*

Fir Needle *Abies alba, Abies sachalinensis, Abies sibirica*

Fragonia *Agonis fragrans*

Frankincense *Boswellia carteri, Boswellia frereana*

Geranium *Pelargonium graveolens*

Ginger *Zingiber officinale*

Grapefruit *Citrus x paradisi*

Helichrysum *Helichrysum italicum, Helichrysum splendidum*

Jasmine *absolute Jasminum sambac*

Juniper berry *Juniperus communis*

Lavender *Lavandula angustifolia*

Lavender, Spike *Lavandula latifolia*

Lemon *Citrus x limon*

Lemon Eucalyptus *Eucalyptus citriodora*

Steam-Distilled Lime *Citrus x aurantifolia*

Marjoram, Sweet *Marjorana hortensis*

Mandarin *Citrus reticulata*

Neroli *Citrus x aurantium*

Orange, Sweet *Citrus sinensis*

Palmarosa *Cymbopogon martinii var motia*

Patchouli *Pogostemon cablin*

Petitgrain *Citrus aurantium*

Pine, Scots *Pinus sylvestris*

Rosalina *Melaleuca ericifolia*

Rose, Otto *Rosa damascena*

Rosewood *Aniba rosaeodora*

Sandalwood *Santalum spicatum*

Spearmint *Mentha spicata*

Spruce, Norway *Picea abies*

Tangerine *Citrus reticulata*

Tea Tree *Melaleuca alternifolia*

Thyme ct linalool *Thymus vulgaris*

Vanilla 12% CO2 Extract *Vanilla planfolia*

Vetiver *Vetiveria zizanoides*

Ylang Ylang *Cananga odorata*

Essential Oils Safe for Babies 3+ Months

The following essential oils are safe to use with three-month-olds and older babies. These gentleessential oils will be the first oils you test on baby.

Chamomile, Roman/German *Anthemis nobilis, Matricaria rectutita*

Dill weed *Anthum graveolens*

Lavender *Lavendula angustifolia*

Rosalina *Melaleuca ericifolia*

Sweet Orange *Citrus sinensis*

Essential Oils Safe for Babies 6+ Months

The following essential oils are safe for use on six-month olds. Babies this age can also use the essential oils listed in the previous list for 3+ month old babies.

Bergamot *Citrus bergamia*

Blue Tansy *Tanacetum annuum*

Carrot Seed *Daucus carota*

Cedarwood, Atlas/Virginia *Cedrus atlantica, Cedrus deodora, Juniperus virginiana*

Cinnamon leaf *Cinnamomum verum*

Citronella *Cymbopogon nardus*

Coriander *Coriandrum sativum*

Cypress *Cupressus sempervires*

Fir needle *Abies sibirica*

Geranium *Pelargonium graveolens*

Grapefruit *Citrus paradisi*

Helichrysum *Helichrysum angustifolium, Helichrysum italicum*

Lemon *Citrus limon*

Marjoram *Marjorana hortensis*

Mandarin *Citrus reticulata*

Neroli *Citrus aurantium*

Palma Rosa *Cymbopogon martinii*

Petitgrain *Citrus aurantium*

Pine *pinus divaricata, pinus resinosa, pinus strobus, pinus sylvestris*

Ravensara *Ravensara aromatica*

Rose Otto *Rosa damascena*

Sandalwood *Santalum spicatum*

Spruce *picea abies, picea glauca, picea mariana, picea rubens*

Tangerine *Citrus reticulata*

Tea Tree *Melaleuca alternifolia*

Essential Oils Safe for Children 2+ Years

The following essential oils are safe for use on children 2+ years. Children this age can also use the essential oils listed for the previous ages.

Basil, Lemon *Ociumum x citriodorum*

Basil, Sweet *Ocimum basilicum*

Benzoin *Styrax benzoin, Styrax paralleloneurus*

Black Pepper *Piper nigrum*

Clary Sage *Salvia sclarea*

Clove Bud/Clove Leaf *Syzygium aromaticum, Eugenia aromatica, Eugenia caryophyllata*

Copaiba Basalm *Copaifera officinalis*

Frankincense *Boswellia carterii*

Ginger *Zingiber officinale*

Hyssop *Hyssopus officinalis*

Juniper Berry *Juniperus communis*

Lemongrass *Andropogon citratus, Andropogon flexuosus, Cymbopogon citratus, Cymbopogon flexuosus*

Lime *Citrus x aurantifolia*

Melissa/Lemon Balm *Melissa officinalis*

Myrrh *Commiphora myrrha*

Oregano *Origanum onites, Origanum smyrnaeum, Origanum vulgare, Origanum compactum, Origanum hirtum, Thymbra capitata, Thymus capitatus, Coridothymus capitatus, Satureeja capitata*

Patchouli *Pogostemon cablin*

Spearmint *Mentha cardiaca, Mentha spicata*

Tea Tree, Lemon *Leptospermum petersonii, Leptospermum citratum, Leptospermum liversidgei*

Thyme *Thymus vulgaris, Thymus Zygis*

Tumeric *Curcuma longa*

Verbena, Lemon *Aloysia triphylla, Aloysia citriodora, Lippa citriodora, Lippa triphylla*

Vetiver *Vetiveria zizanoides*

Valerian *Valeriana officinalis*

Ylang Ylang *Cananga odorata*

Essential Oils Safe for Children 6+ Years

The following essential oils are safe for use on children 6+ years. Children this age can also use the essential oils listed for the previous ages. It is now safe to use all the same essential oils that adults use, in moderation.

Anise/Aniseed *Pimpinella anisum*

Anise, Star *Illicium verum*

Cajeput *Melaleuca cajuputi, Melaleuca leucadendron*

Cardamom *Elettaria cardamomum*

Cornmint *Mentha arvensis, Mentha canadensis*

Eucalyptus *Eucalyptus camaldulensis, Eucalyptus globulus, Eucalyptus maidenii, Eucalyptus plenissima, Eucalyptus kochii, Eucalyptus polybractea, Eucalyptus radiata, Eucalyptus autraliana, Eucalyptus phellandra, Eucalyptus smithii*

Fennel, sweet and bitter *Foeniculum vulgare*

Laurel Leaf/Bay Laurel *Laurus nobilis*

Marjoram, Spanish *Thymus mastichina*

Niaouli *cineole chemotype*

Nutmeg *Myristica fragrans*

Peppermint *Mentha x piperita*

Rosemary *Rosmarinus officinalis*

Sage *Salvia officinalis, Salvia fruiticosa, Salvia tribola, Salvia apiana*

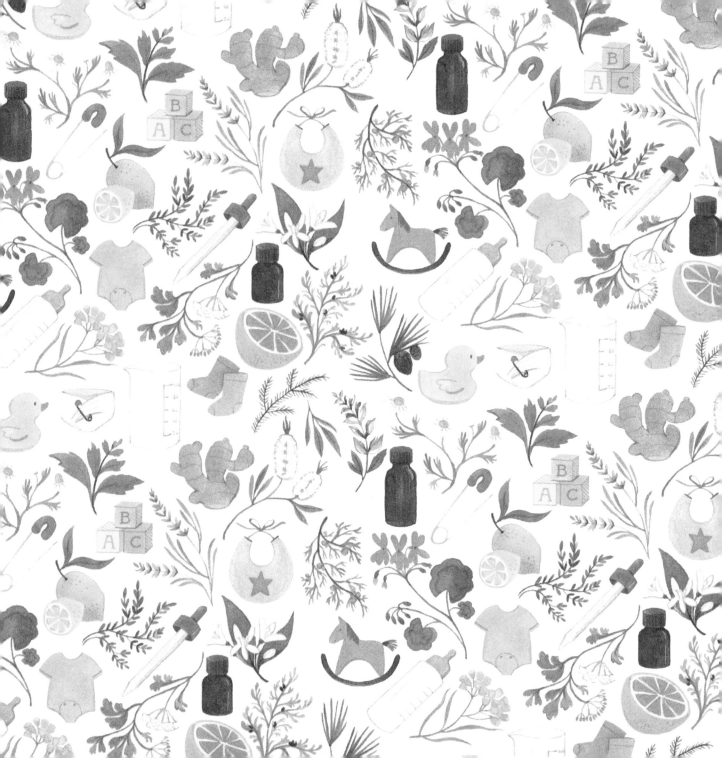

PART 2

Essential Oil Blends & Remedies

You can do so much more with essential oils than adding a few drops of your favorite one to a diffuser. In this part, I offer a number of remedies for the most common ailments that arise during pregnancy and beyond. You'll find two to three unique recipes for each ailment, all including essential oils. Chapter 3 is dedicated to pregnancy and the many issues that may arise during your pregnancy, everything from morning sickness to stretch marks. Chapter 4 is all about labor, delivery, and breastfeeding mamas. Create birthing room sprays, anxiety-relieving diffuser blends, and even a nipple cream that you will thank me for if you choose to breast-feed your child. With over 100 remedies created with babies and children in mind, chapter 5 focuses on the many ailments and issues that arise when raising little ones. Each remedy will specify safe dilutions for each age range and will even offer substitution and safety tips, so that you can safely customize each recipe for you and your children. All of the remedies in this book will also specify the method of application (topical or inhaled) and will warn you of photosensitizing essential oils ahead of time, so that you can be sure to avoid sunlight when needed. All recipes in this book are made using essential oils that are safe for use around both adults and children, so that you can be sure using a blend in the diffuser or on yourself topically will not harm your little ones in the process.

A NOTE ON TOOLS AND EQUIPMENT

If you are new to essential oils, you may need to stock your cabinet with a few tools and utensils that you will need when making many of the recipes in this book. While there are all kinds of fun essential oil tools out there, you don't need all of them to get started on your natural aromatherapeutic journey, but to get the most out of this book, you will need at least the following:

DIFFUSERS A good diffuser is a must in aromatherapy. There are quite a few different styles that you can purchase, but I prefer ultrasonic diffusers. With the ultrasonic diffuser, you add water to a fill line, and then add the essential oils to the water. The diffuser uses ultrasonic vibrations to disperse the water vapor and essential oils into the air all around the room. I recommend purchasing diffusers that have different timed on/off settings that make overexposure easy to avoid.

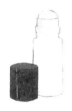

GLASS ROLL-ON BOTTLES (⅓-OUNCE) Roll-on bottles are great for applying topical essential oils. I always keep a lot of these around and even reuse them.

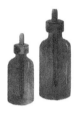

DARK GLASS ESSENTIAL OIL BOTTLES While you can purchase these bottles new, the best and cheapest way to acquire these bottles is to save the bottles your essential oils originally came in. Clean them out by filling them with salt, then rinsing them clean. Remember, undiluted essential oils and essential oil blends must be stored in dark glass bottles. Plastic is never advised for storing undiluted essential oils, because the oils can degrade the plastic.

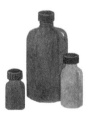

STORAGE AND DELIVERY RECEPTACLES When making your own healing remedies, all sorts of different storage containers are needed to house your creations. Depending on what you are creating, you may need a spray bottle, a small metal tin, a glass jar, or even a lotion pump bottle to keep your creations in. You can find many of these containers online, but I also like to recycle all of the containers from the cosmetic products I purchase. Don't forget to sterilize them first! I often use the dishwasher to sterilize old shampoo bottles, lotion bottles, spray bottles, and even lip balm containers.

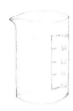

LIQUID MEASURING CUP If you have ever tried to measure liquids in measuring spoons and cups, you have likely experienced the mess of trying to pour those liquids into a container. My life was changed forever when I discovered the beaker-like liquid measuring cups. There are also smaller versions that measure out ounces and tablespoons.

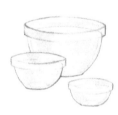

GLASS BOWLS Undiluted essential oils will degrade plastic and can even strip paint off a container. I suggest using glass bowls when mixing up your essential oil creations. Metal bowls can also be used, but I avoid using metal with bentonite clay-based products, because it reacts with and reduces the healing effectiveness of the clay. Glass bowls are usually best.

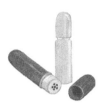

AROMATHERAPY INHALERS Just like roll-on bottles, aromatherapy inhalers are very cheap and easy to acquire. I love them because of their discreet and personal nature. They are great to keep in your purse or diaper bag, so you can pull them out whenever the need arises.

UNDERSTANDING MEDICINAL PROPERTIES

You'll see several primarily medicinal terms peppered throughout the rest of the book in descriptions of remedies of plant profiles. While some, such as *antidepressant*, might be obvious, you might never have heard of others, such as *carminative*. Turn to page 261 for a mini glossary of important terms you'll see again and again in this book.

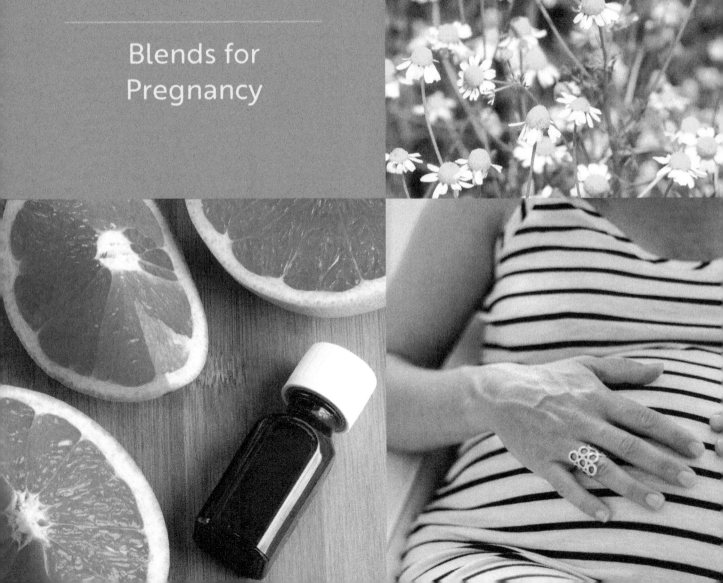

CHAPTER
THREE

Blends for Pregnancy

Acne

Because of hormonal changes, pregnancy can increase acne and blemishes on your face and body. If you don't already have a facial cleaning regimen in place, starting one now can help fend off most acne problems. Always cleanse your face twice a day, followed by a toner to close pores, and finish with a moisturizer to lock the moisture into your skin. Essential oils can be very helpful when it comes to cleansing and healing the skin. Those excellent for acne-prone skin include lavender, tea tree, rosalina, palmarosa, sweet orange, cedarwood, cypress, geranium, and chamomile oils.

ZIPPY ZIT ZAPPER SPOT TREATMENT
MAKES 1 OUNCE ➢ TOPICAL ➢ PHOTOSENSITIZING

2 tablespoons hemp seed oil

5 drops grapefruit essential oil

5 drops lavender essential oil

3 drops tea tree essential oil

1. Add all the ingredients to a dark glass bottle, and swirl to combine.

2. Using a cotton swab, apply treatment to blemishes after cleansing your face. Apply before using toner or moisturizer, or, if using makeup, allow 5 minutes for the treatment to sink in before applying.

AWESOME ADDITION Hemp seed oil is one of my favorite carrier oils for acne-prone skin, but grapeseed oil is also wonderful for fighting blemishes. I like to add both hemp seed and grapeseed oil to this recipe!

MOISTURIZING FACIAL OIL FOR ACNE-PRONE SKIN
MAKES 1 OUNCE ➢ TOPICAL ➢ PHOTOSENSITIZING

1 tablespoon hemp seed oil

½ tablespoon jojoba oil

½ tablespoon grapeseed oil

3 drops lavender essential oil

3 drops palmarosa essential oil

1 drop steam-distilled lemon essential oil

1. Add all the ingredients to a bottle with a dropper or lotion pump and swirl to combine.

2. Cleanse and tone your face.

3. Dispense 1 to 3 drops of moisturizing oil onto your palm, rub palms together, and massage the oil into your face. I personally use 1 drop of oil for my morning application and 2 to 3 drops of oil for my evening application.

CAUTION Cold-pressed lemon essential oil is photosensitizing and can cause a rash at the application site when exposed to sunlight. I suggest using steam-distilled lemon essential oil in this recipe, since this blend is meant for daily use.

MOISTURIZING FACIAL TONER FOR ACNE-PRONE SKIN
MAKES 4 OUNCES ≫ TOPICAL

¼ cup witch hazel
1 teaspoon vegetable glycerin
2 teaspoons aloe vera gel
5 drops lavender essential oil

5 drops sweet orange essential oil
3 drops Atlas cedarwood essential oil
Filtered water

1. Add all the ingredients to a 4-ounce spray bottle. Add enough filtered water to fill the bottle, and swirl to combine.
2. Cleanse your face. Spray the toner onto your clean face, and follow with a moisturizer.

STORAGE Store in a cool, dark location for 6 to 9 months. You can keep this in the refrigerator for a longer shelf life (9 to 12 months).

SUBSTITUTION TIP For even more moisturizing and healing properties, substitute the water in this recipe with a hydrosol. My favorites to use? Chamomile or calendula.

Allergies

Seasonal allergies can strike any time of year. Many people turn to eucalyptus for sinus and allergy relief, but eucalyptus should be avoided during pregnancy. A member of the same family as tea tree, rosalina is my favorite pregnancy and kid-safe antiseptic essential oil. It opens up sinuses, reduces inflammation, and helps soothe irritated mucous membranes. German chamomile is another gentle essential oil for allergies and hay fever because of azulene, the chemical constituent that gives it its blue color and acts as a natural antihistamine.

ALLERGY INHALER BLEND
MAKES 1 TREATMENT ↣ AROMATIC

15 drops rosalina essential oil
10 drops sweet orange essential oil

5 drops German chamomile essential oil

1. Combine all the essential oils in a small glass bowl.
2. Using tweezers, add the wick (the cotton pad) of an aromatherapy personal inhaler to the bowl and roll it around until it's soaked up all of the essential oils mixture.
3. Use the tweezers to transfer the wick to the inhaler tube. Close the tube and label the inhaler.
4. Take a whiff of the inhaler whenever seasonal allergies affect you.

SUBSTITUTION TIP You can substitute blue tansy essential oil for German chamomile. Blue tansy is safe to use for babies or while pregnant. It contains azulene, the same constituent that gives German chamomile essential oil its blue color.

HAY FEVER DIFFUSER BLEND
MAKES ½ OUNCE ↣ AROMATIC

1 teaspoon rosalina essential oil
¾ teaspoon fir needle essential oil

¾ teaspoon lavender essential oil
45 drops lemon essential oil

1. Add all the essential oils to an empty essential oil bottle (or any dark glass bottle with a dropper), and gently swirl to combine.
2. Add 10 drops to a diffuser and diffuse throughout the room in 10 to 15 minute increments (10 to 15 minutes on/30 minutes off) to avoid overexposure.

HELPFUL HINT To make an aromatherapy inhaler, follow the instructions for the Allergy Inhaler Blend (page 38) and substitute 30 drops of this blend for the essential oils in the recipe.

ALLERGY SALT STEAM
MAKES 1 TREATMENT ↣ AROMATIC

2 drops frankincense essential oil
2 drops lavender essential oil

2 drops sweet orange essential oil
¼ cup sea salt

1. In a small glass bowl, mix together all the ingredients until the oils are distributed evenly.
2. Bring 4 to 6 cups of water to a boil. Add the salt mixture to a large bowl.
3. Pour the boiling water over the salt mixture and mix together until the salt dissolves.
4. Cover your head with a towel and position your face over the bowl, using the towel as a tent to keep the steam in.
5. With your eyes closed and face 5 to 10 inches away from the hot water, breathe in the steam for no more than 10 minutes at a time.

Anxiety

With today's busy lifestyles, many women experience stress and anxiety throughout their pregnancy—whether it's their first baby or last—and that's completely natural. It's important to take time for yourself to relax. You might try meditation, yoga, or light walks in nature to help relieve stress and anxiety. Essential oils helpful at relieving life's stressors include lavender, chamomile, lemon, sweet orange, grapefruit, coriander, bergamot, vanilla, sandalwood, ylang-ylang, cedarwood, and neroli.

DON'T WORRY BE HAPPY ROLL-ON
MAKES ⅓ OUNCE ≫ TOPICAL ≫ PHOTOSENSITIZING

1 drop grapefruit essential oil
1 drop Roman chamomile essential oil

1 drop sweet orange essential oil
Fractionated coconut oil

1. Add the grapefruit, Roman chamomile, and sweet orange essential oils to a ⅓-ounce glass roll-on bottle.
2. Add enough coconut oil to fill the bottle. Place the roller ball and cap on and gently swirl to combine. Don't forget to label your creation.
3. Roll the blend onto the back of your neck, chest, and wrists whenever you are feeling anxious or stressed.

SUBSTITUTION TIP If you don't have chamomile essential oil on hand, lavender essential oil can be substituted in this recipe.

ANTI-ANXIETY DIFFUSER BLEND

MAKES ½ OUNCE ⇒ TOPICAL ⇒ AROMATIC ⇒ PHOTOSENSITIZING

1 teaspoon bergamot essential oil

¾ teaspoon grapefruit essential oil

¾ teaspoon lavender essential oil

½ teaspoon coriander essential oil

1. Add all the essential oils to an empty essential oil bottle (or any dark glass bottle with a dropper) and gently swirl to combine.
2. Add 10 drops to a diffuser and diffuse throughout the room in 10 to 15 minute increments (10 to 15 minutes on/30 minutes off) to avoid overexposure.

HELPFUL HINT This essential oil blend can be used in a massage oil or even your favorite unscented lotion. Simply add 8 or 9 drops of this blend to 1 ounce of oil or lotion and mix to combine. Remember that both bergamot and grapefruit essential oils can cause photosensitization, so always dilute this blend when using on your skin, and use extra caution in the sun.

ROOM SPRAY FOR ANXIETY

MAKES 6 OUNCES ⇒ AROMATIC

25 drops bergamot essential oil

20 drops lavender essential oil

15 drops neroli essential oil

2 tablespoons 80-proof vodka

5 ounces filtered water

1. Add all the ingredients to a spray bottle and shake to combine.
2. Spray around the room and on pillows and furniture.

Backaches

Having had more back surgeries in the first twenty years of my life than most people do in a lifetime, I am a pro at soothing a sore back. There are many reasons your back might be aching, including injury, slipped disc, arthritis, or even just the weight of your baby bump, but most backaches can be relieved using essential oils. Some of my favorite essential oils used for back pain relief are lavender, rosalina, marjoram, fir needle, cypress, juniper berry, helichrysum, chamomile, black pepper, and spearmint.

ANTI-INFLAMMATORY SALVE

MAKES 4 OUNCES ❧ TOPICAL

¼ cup plus 2 tablespoons unrefined coconut oil

2 tablespoons beeswax pastilles

10 drops lavender essential oil

10 drops rosalina essential oil

8 drops fir needle essential oil

8 drops marjoram essential oil

1. In a small pan over low heat, melt the coconut oil and beeswax.

2. Once melted, remove from heat and stir in the lavender, rosalina, fir needle, and marjoram essential oils.

3. Pour the mixture into a Mason jar, and put into the freezer for 20 minutes to harden.

4. To use, apply a dime-size amount of the salve to the aching area and massage it in.

5. Store in a cool, dark location.

AWESOME ADDITION For the best back pain relief possible, steep 2 tablespoons arnica flowers in the melted coconut oil over low heat for 1 hour. Strain off, then continue with the recipe.

BACK MASSAGE OIL

MAKES 4 OUNCES ❧ TOPICAL

½ cup coconut oil

10 drops marjoram essential oil

10 drops rosalina essential oil

8 drops coriander essential oil

8 drops spearmint essential oil

1. In a small pan over low heat, melt the coconut oil.

2. Once melted, remove from heat, add the marjoram, rosalina, coriander, and spearmint essential oils, and stir to combine.

3. Pour into a Mason jar, and put into the freezer for 20 minutes to harden.

4. To use, apply a small amount of the salve to the affected areas and massage it in.

5. Store in a cool, dark location.

SOOTHE YOUR BACKACHE BATH
MAKES 1 TREATMENT ≫ TOPICAL

5 drops lavender essential oil
3 drops Roman chamomile essential oil
2 drops helichrysum essential oil

1 tablespoon unscented shampoo or
   liquid castile soap
1 cup Epsom salt

1. In a small bowl, stir together the lavender, chamomile, and helichrysum essential oils with the shampoo or liquid soap.

2. Place the Epsom salt in a medium bowl and stir in the soap mixture.

3. Pour the mixture under the running bath water as you fill the tub.

SUBSTITUTION TIP Instead of unscented soap, you can alternately use your favorite carrier oil in this recipe, but be cautious when exiting because the oil will make the tub very slippery.

Breast Tenderness

For many women, breast tenderness is one of the first signs that they are pregnant. Unfortunately for me, it lasted throughout my entire pregnancy, but I found great relief from massages using lavender and marjoram essential oils. Other essential oils that are very helpful at relieving the pain of breast tenderness are chamomile, ylang-ylang, grapefruit, rosalina, geranium, frankincense, and helichrysum.

SOOTHING BREAST MASSAGE OIL
MAKES 2 OUNCES ≫ TOPICAL

2 tablespoons unrefined coconut oil
8 drops lavender essential oil

6 drops marjoram essential oil
4 drops cypress essential oil

1. In a small pan over low heat, melt the coconut oil.

2. Once melted, remove from heat, add the lavender, marjoram, and cypress essential oils, and stir to combine.

3. Pour into a Mason jar and store in a cool, dark location.

4. To use, massage a small amount into your breasts whenever painful and tender.

ANTI-INFLAMMATORY BOOBIE BALM

MAKES 4 OUNCES ❧ TOPICAL

¼ cup plus 2 tablespoons unrefined coconut oil

2 tablespoons beeswax pastilles

16 drops lavender essential oil

12 drops rosalina essential oil

8 drops German chamomile essential oil

1. In a small pan over low heat, melt the coconut oil and beeswax.

2. Once melted, remove from heat and add the lavender, rosalina, and chamomile essential oils.

3. Pour into a Mason jar, and put into the freezer for 20 minutes to harden. Store in a cool, dark location.

4. To use, apply a dime-size amount to your breasts and massage in.

SUBSTITUTION TIP If you don't have German chamomile essential oil on hand, you can substitute Roman chamomile or geranium essential oils.

Carpal Tunnel Syndrome

Oddly enough, carpal tunnel syndrome (also called median nerve compression) is a common problem for women during pregnancy. If you didn't already have this condition to begin with, it may occur during pregnancy due to increased fluid retention putting extra pressure on the median nerve. Carpal tunnel from pregnancy usually goes away on its own, but in the meantime there are essential oils (lavender, ginger, marjoram, rosalina, spearmint, turmeric CO_2, cypress, frankincense, and helichrysum) that can help relieve the pain and pressure.

GINGER PAIN-RELIEVING SALVE

MAKES 4 OUNCES ⇒ TOPICAL

¼ cup plus 2 tablespoons extra-virgin olive oil

2 tablespoons beeswax pastilles

20 drops ginger essential oil

10 drops lavender essential oil

6 drops marjoram essential oil

1. In a small pan over low heat, heat the olive oil and beeswax.
2. Once melted, remove from heat and add the ginger, lavender, and marjoram essential oils.
3. Pour into a Mason jar, and put into the freezer for 20 minutes to harden. Store in a cool, dark location.
4. To use, apply a dime-size amount of the salve to the aching area and massage it in.

AWESOME ADDITION To enhance the effectiveness of this salve, steep 2 tablespoons St. John's wort in the olive oil over low heat for 1 hour. Strain off, then continue with the recipe. St. John's wort is known for its natural ability to reduce inflammation and relieve pain, including nerve pain.

CARPAL TUNNEL MASSAGE OIL

MAKES 4 OUNCES ⇒ TOPICAL

½ cup unrefined coconut oil

16 drops cypress essential oil

14 drops lavender essential oil

6 drops turmeric CO_2 essential oil

1. In a small pan over low heat, melt the coconut oil.
2. Once melted, remove from heat, add the cypress, lavender, and turmeric CO_2 essential oils, and stir to combine.
3. Pour into a Mason jar, and put into the freezer for 20 minutes to harden. Store in a cool, dark location.
4. To use, apply a small amount of the oil to the area that aches and massage it in.

AWESOME ADDITION To enhance the effectiveness of this massage oil, steep 2 to 4 tablespoons cayenne powder in the coconut oil over low heat for 1 hour. Strain off, and continue with the recipe. Cayenne is a fantastic analgesic and helps get the circulation moving.

Constipation

With all of the hormone changes that happen during pregnancy, constipation is a common problem. Drinking plenty of water and eating lots of fresh fruits and vegetables will help keep things moving along regularly, but essential oils can also aid in relieving some of the pain and gas that come along with constipation. Some essential oils that help with constipation are dill weed, chamomile, spearmint, ginger, sweet orange, lemon, frankincense, petitgrain, and coriander.

ABDOMINAL MASSAGE OIL #1
MAKES 4 OUNCES ⇒ TOPICAL

½ cup unrefined coconut oil
20 drops sweet orange essential oil

10 drops Roman chamomile essential oil
6 drops dill weed essential oil

1. In a small pan over low heat, melt the coconut oil.
2. Once melted, remove from heat, add the sweet orange, Roman chamomile, and dill weed essential oils, and stir to combine.
3. Pour into a Mason jar, and put into the freezer for 20 minutes to harden. Store in a cool, dark location.
4. To use, apply a small amount to your abdomen and massage in.

ABDOMINAL MASSAGE OIL #2
MAKES 4 OUNCES ⇒ TOPICAL

½ cup unrefined coconut oil
16 drops sweet orange essential oil

10 drops black pepper essential oil
10 drops ginger essential oil

1. In a small pan over low heat, melt the coconut oil.
2. Once melted, remove from heat, add the sweet orange, black pepper, and ginger essential oils, and stir to combine.
3. Pour into a Mason jar, and put into the freezer for 20 minutes to harden. Store in a cool, dark location when not in use.
4. To use, apply a small amount to your abdomen and massage in.

DIGESTIVE SALVE
MAKES 4 OUNCES ❧ TOPICAL

¼ cup plus 2 tablespoons unrefined
   coconut oil
2 tablespoons beeswax pastilles
10 drops ginger essential oil

10 drops Roman chamomile essential oil
10 drops spearmint essential oil
6 drops black pepper essential oil

1. In a small pan over low heat, melt the coconut oil and beeswax.
2. Once melted, remove from heat, add the ginger, Roman chamomile, spearmint, and black pepper essential oils, and stir to combine.
3. Pour into a Mason jar, and put into the freezer for 20 minutes to harden. Store in a cool, dark location.
4. To use, apply a dime-size amount to your abdomen and massage in.

Cold and Flu

If you have a cold or the flu you may be experiencing all sorts of symptoms, such as fever, chills, body aches, cough, sore throat, runny noses, congestion, and more. Because many of the symptoms for cold and flu are similar, they can be treated with the same remedies. Peppered throughout the chapter are recipes for coughs, congestion, and aches and pains, so here, you will find recipes for killing germs in your home, a cold and flu bath remedy, and a fever-reducing compress. There are many essential oils helpful for cold and flu, including lavender, tea tree, fir needle, cypress, juniper berry, spearmint, rosalina, marjoram, frankincense, chamomile, spruce, all citrus, palmarosa, blue tansy, and pine.

ANTI-GERM DIFFUSER BLEND
MAKES ½ OUNCE ❧ AROMATIC

1 teaspoon rosalina essential oil
¾ teaspoon lavender essential oil

¾ teaspoon marjoram essential oil
½ teaspoon fir needle essential oil

1. Add all the essential oils to an empty essential oil bottle (or any dark glass bottle with a dropper) and gently swirl to combine.

2. Add 10 drops to a diffuser and diffuse throughout the room in 10 to 15 minute increments (10 to 15 minutes on/30 minutes off) to avoid overexposure.

HELPFUL HINT Add this essential oil blend to a humidifier or dilute in coconut oil before rubbing on your chest and body. Always dilute before using topically.

HEALING BATH
MAKES 1 TREATMENT ≫ TOPICAL ≫ AROMATIC

5 drops rosalina essential oil
3 drops frankincense essential oil
3 drops lavender essential oil

1 tablespoon unscented shampoo or liquid castile soap
1 cup Epsom salt

1. In a small bowl, stir together the rosalina, frankincense, and lavender essential oils with the shampoo or liquid soap.
2. Place the Epsom salt in a medium bowl and stir in the soap mixture.
3. Pour the mixture under the running bath water as you fill the tub.

SUBSTITUTION TIP Instead of unscented soap, you can alternately use your favorite carrier oil in this recipe, but be cautious when exiting because the oil will make the tub very slippery.

FEVER-REDUCING COOLING COMPRESS
MAKES 1 TREATMENT ≫ TOPICAL ≫ AROMATIC

5 drops spearmint essential oil
3 drops fir needle essential oil
2 drops lemon essential oil

1 tablespoon aloe vera gel
2 tablespoons raw apple cider vinegar
4 cups cool water

1. In a small bowl, stir together the spearmint, fir needle, and lemon essential oils with the aloe vera gel.
2. In a medium bowl, stir together the vinegar, water, and aloe vera mixture.
3. To use, dip a washcloth into the remedy and squeeze off any excess. Apply to the forehead and feet to help draw heat from the body.

SUBSTITUTION TIP You can substitute peppermint tea for the water here. Steep ½ cup peppermint leaves in 4 cups boiling water for 15 to 20 minutes, then add just enough ice cubes to bring the tea's temperature down to cool—not cold—temperature.

Cough

Not all coughs are created equal. There are two different types of coughs, dry and wet coughs, and each requires a different approach. Dry coughs can be identified by their intense bouts of spastic coughing and/or a tickling of the throat, while wet coughs are easily identified with the constant production of mucus and phlegm. Dry coughs require remedies to calm and sooth the cough, while the phlegm produced by wet coughs should be expelled. Some of my favorite essential oils that work well at soothing a cough and getting rid of the phlegm include lavender, tea tree, rosalina, fir needle, cypress, pine, juniper berry, frankincense, chamomile, spearmint, blue tansy, and lemon.

DRY COUGH CHEST RUB

MAKES 4 OUNCES ⤳ TOPICAL ⤳ AROMATIC

½ cup unrefined coconut oil
10 drops fir needle essential oil
10 drops lavender essential oil

10 drops marjoram essential oil
6 drops spearmint essential oil

1. In a small pan over low heat, melt the coconut oil.
2. Once melted, remove from heat, add the fir needle, lavender, marjoram, and spearmint essential oils, and stir to combine.
3. Pour into a Mason jar, and put into the freezer for 20 minutes to harden.
4. Store in a cool, dark location.
5. Rub onto your chest, back, and the bottoms of your feet. Cover the feet with socks immediately after application.

EXPECTORANT CHEST RUB

MAKES 4 OUNCES ⤳ TOPICAL ⤳ AROMATIC

½ cup unrefined coconut oil
10 drops cypress essential oil
10 drops frankincense essential oil

10 drops lavender essential oil
6 drops tea tree essential oil

1. In a small pan over low heat, melt the coconut oil.

2. Once melted, remove from heat, add the cypress, frankincense, lavender, and tea tree essential oils, and stir to combine.

3. Pour into a Mason jar, and put into the freezer for 20 minutes to harden. Store in a cool, dark location.

4. To use, rub on your chest, back, and the bottoms of your feet. Cover the feet with socks immediately after application.

SOOTHE YOUR COUGH DIFFUSER BLEND
MAKES ½ OUNCE ➤ AROMATIC

1 teaspoon fir needle essential oil

1 teaspoon rosalina essential oil

½ teaspoon cypress essential oil

½ teaspoon lavender essential oil

1. Add all the essential oils to an empty essential oil bottle (or any dark glass bottle with a dropper), and gently swirl the bottle to combine.

2. Add 10 drops to a diffuser and diffuse throughout the room in 10 to 15 minute increments (10 to 15 minutes on/30 minutes off) to avoid overexposure.

Depression

Anyone can experience depression during and after pregnancy. It is important to be mindful of your emotional state, and tell someone how you are feeling. Essential oils have had a track record of being able to lighten moods, reduce stress and anger, and even help relax tension from the body. My favorite essential oils to use for depression include lavender, chamomile, neroli, sandalwood, ylang-ylang, grapefruit, sweet orange, bergamot, frankincense, geranium, and marjoram.

ANTIDEPRESSANT DIFFUSER BLEND #1

MAKES ½ OUNCE ⤳ AROMATIC ⤳ PHOTOSENSITIZING

1¼ teaspoons grapefruit essential oil
1¼ teaspoons sweet orange essential oil
25 drops neroli essential oil
25 drops ylang-ylang essential oil

1. Add all the essential oils to an empty essential oil bottle (or any dark glass bottle with a dropper) and gently swirl the bottle to combine.
2. Add 10 drops to a diffuser and diffuse throughout the room in 10 to 15 minute increments (10 to 15 minutes on/30 minutes off) to avoid overexposure.

HELPFUL HINT This essential oil blend can be added to your favorite lotion or diluted in coconut oil to rub on your chest and body. Since the blend is very strong, don't forget to dilute before using topically, and remember that grapefruit oil causes photosensitization, so use caution in the sun.

ANTIDEPRESSANT DIFFUSER BLEND #2

MAKES ½ OUNCE ⤳ AROMATIC

1 teaspoon marjoram essential oil
¾ teaspoon lavender essential oil
¾ teaspoon tangerine essential oil
½ teaspoon frankincense essential oil

1. Add all the essential oils to an empty essential oil bottle (or any dark glass bottle with a dropper) and gently swirl the bottle to combine.
2. Add 10 drops to a diffuser and diffuse throughout the room in 10 to 15 minute increments (10 to 15 minutes on/30 minutes off) to avoid overexposure.

SUBSTITUTION TIP If you don't have tangerine essential oil on hand, any other citrus essential oil will work in its place. My favorites are sweet orange or bergamot.

HAPPY MAMA AROMATHERAPY INHALER

MAKES 1 TREATMENT ⤳ AROMATIC

1 teaspoon bergamot essential oil
1 teaspoon lemon essential oil
¾ teaspoon coriander essential oil
25 drops ylang-ylang essential oil

1. Combine all the essential oils in a small glass bowl.

2. Using tweezers, add the wick (the cotton pad) of an aromatherapy personal inhaler to the bowl, and roll it around until it's soaked up all of the essential oils mixture.

3. Use the tweezers to transfer the wick to the inhaler tube. Close the tube and label the inhaler.

4. Take a whiff of the inhaler whenever you need a ray of sunshine and happiness.

Dizziness

Dizziness can strike at any moment, leaving a pregnant mama unsteady and off balance. Rising hormones causes blood vessels to relax, which lowers blood pressure, causing dizziness. Lavender, spearmint, lemon, sweet orange, grapefruit, rosalina, chamomile, cypress, fir needle, frankincense, ginger, and juniper berry essential oils can help settle your equilibrium, wake up your senses, and get the flow of circulation going again.

KEEPIN' IT STEADY AROMATHERAPY INHALER
MAKES 1 TREATMENT ⇒ AROMATIC

15 drops sweet orange essential oil
10 drops spearmint essential oil

5 drops lemon essential oil

1. Combine all the essential oils in a small glass bowl.

2. Using tweezers, add the wick (the cotton pad) of an aromatherapy personal inhaler to the bowl and roll it around until it's soaked up all of the essential oils mixture.

3. Use the tweezers to transfer the wick to the inhaler tube. Close the tube and label the inhaler.

4. Take a whiff of the inhaler whenever dizziness occurs.

MAKES 1 TREATMENT ﹥ AROMATIC

7 drops lemon essential oil

5 drops rosalina essential oil

3 drops spearmint essential oil

Fine or course sea salt

1. In a ⅓-ounce glass bottle, add the lemon, rosalina, and spearmint essential oils.

2. Fill the remainder of the bottle with the sea salt.

3. Waft the bottle under your nose while taking deep inhalations whenever you feel a dizzy spell coming on.

SAFETY TIP Overexposure to essential oils can cause headaches and dizziness. Avoid exposure to essential oils for more than 30 minutes at a time.

Ear Infection

It is a common misconception that antibiotics should be given at the first sign of an ear infection. Most ear infections are viral, not bacterial, making the antibiotic prescription worthless. Even the Centers for Disease Control has agreed, saying: "Ear infections will often get better on their own without antibiotic treatment." And many studies have shown that using antibiotics unnecessarily can be harmful. Essential oils such as lavender, chamomile, rosalina, palmarosa, tea tree, marjoram, and frankincense can help reduce inflammation and soothe pain caused by an ear infection, while aiding your body in fighting the virus.

SOOTHING GARLIC EAR OIL

MAKES 4 OUNCES ﹥ TOPICAL

½ cup extra-virgin olive oil

3 garlic cloves, minced

9 drops lavender essential oil

3 drops palmarosa essential oil

3 drops rosalina essential oil

1. In a small pan over low heat, combine the olive oil and garlic. Steep the garlic in the oil over low heat for 1 to 3 hours.

2. Remove the pan from the heat. Using a fine mesh sieve or cheesecloth, strain the oil into a glass bowl taking great care not to leave any garlic in the strained oil.

3. Add the lavender, palmarosa, and rosalina essential oils, and swirl gently to combine. Store in a dark glass bottle with a dropper.

4. To use, warm the bottle by either placing it in a bowl of warm water for 3 to 5 minutes, rubbing the bottle between your hands until warm, or running the outside of the dropper under warm water and then quickly drying before sucking up the oil. Be sure to test the oil on your forearm, as you would warmed baby bathwater or milk. Drop 2 to 3 drops of warm oil into each ear every 4 hours as needed. Always treat both ears because ear infections can move from ear to ear.

SAFETY TIP This remedy is not effective for swimmer's ear or other infections caused by water entering the ear; in fact, the remedy can make those types of infections worse. If dealing with a perforated eardrum, do not use this remedy; nothing should be poured into the ear. To be able to know what is going on inside of your child's ear, pick up a Dr. Mom Otoscope (available at DrMomOtoscope.com) for your medicine chest.

EAR AND NECK MASSAGE OIL

MAKES 2 OUNCES ❧ TOPICAL

¼ cup unrefined coconut oil

8 drops lavender essential oil

6 drops rosalina essential oil

4 drops German chamomile essential oil

1. In a small pan over low heat, melt the coconut oil.

2. Once melted, remove from heat, add the lavender, rosalina, and German chamomile essential oils, and stir to combine.

3. Pour into a Mason jar, and put into the freezer for 20 minutes to harden. Store in a cool, dark location.

4. To use, apply a small amount around the ears and neck, massaging in.

Edema and Swelling

During pregnancy, a woman's body produces up to 50 percent more fluids to accommodate the baby growing in the womb. A natural part of pregnancy, edema and swelling are caused by this extra fluid buildup. Essential oils like lavender, cypress, grapefruit, juniper berry, chamomile, ginger, lemon, spearmint, tea tree, geranium, and rosalina can help relieve some of swelling and help to keep your circulation flowing.

SOOTHING FOOT BATH
MAKES 1 TREATMENT ⇒ TOPICAL

1 tablespoon aloe vera gel

4 drops cypress essential oil

2 drops grapefruit essential oil

2 drops lavender essential oil

½ cup Epsom salt

1. In a small bowl, stir together the aloe vera gel with the cypress, grapefruit, and lavender essential oils.
2. Place the Epsom salt in a large mixing bowl and stir in the aloe vera mixture.
3. Pour the water (using your preferred temperature) over the salt mixture and stir until dissolved.
4. Soak your feet in the foot bath for as long as it is comfortable.

CIRCULATORY MASSAGE OIL
MAKES 4 OUNCES ⇒ TOPICAL

½ cup unrefined coconut oil

16 drops ginger essential oil

10 drops lavender essential oil

10 drops lemon essential oil

1. In a small pan over low heat, melt the coconut oil.
2. Once melted, remove from heat, add the ginger, lavender, and lemon essential oils, and stir to combine.
3. Pour into a Mason jar, and put into the freezer for 20 minutes to harden. Store in a cool, dark location.
4. To use, apply a small amount to the swollen area and massage it in.

SOOTHING ANTI-INFLAMMATORY BATH
MAKES 1 TREATMENT → TOPICAL

5 drops lavender essential oil
3 drops cypress essential oil
2 drops lemon essential oil

1 tablespoon unscented shampoo or
    castile soap
1 cup Epsom salt

1. In a small bowl, stir together the lavender, cypress, and lemon essential oils with the shampoo or liquid soap.
2. Place the Epsom salt in a medium bowl and stir in the soap mixture.
3. Pour the mixture under the running bath water as you fill the tub.

AWESOME ADDITION While some essential oils are too strong to use during pregnancy, you can use their whole herb counterparts. Rosemary and nettle are both awesome additions to this anti-inflammatory bath. Add ½ cup of each herb to a cloth tea bag or an old, clean sock, and tie closed before tossing it into the bathtub.

Fetal Positioning

The best position for a smooth birth is with the baby's head pointed down and facing in toward your spine. While there are no guarantees that you will be able to convince the baby to turn, you can try an essential oil massage throughout the third trimester to help ease the baby into the optimal position for birth. When applied to the top of the baby bump, spearmint essential oil causes a cold sensation that is said to stimulate the baby to change positions.

REPOSITIONING MASSAGE OIL #1
MAKES 1 OUNCE → TOPICAL

2 tablespoons unrefined coconut oil

9 drops spearmint essential oil

1. In a small glass bowl, combine the coconut oil and spearmint essential oil.
2. To use, apply over the top of the baby bump, from hip to hip in a rainbow motion.

REPOSITIONING MASSAGE OIL #2

MAKES 1 OUNCE ⤙ TOPICAL

2 tablespoons unrefined coconut oil   9 drops rosalina essential oil

1. In a small glass bowl, combine the coconut oil and rosalina essential oil.

2. To use, apply over the top of the baby bump, from hip to hip in a rainbow motion.

Group B Strep/Bacterial Vaginosis

Group B streptococcus is a vaginal bacterial infection. Found in most people's intestines, the group B streptococcus spreads from there to the vagina for a couple of reasons. (Careful restroom hygiene can decrease spreading of the bacteria.) Group B strep is easily treated using antibacterial herbs and essential oils. Antibacterial essential oils such as lavender, tea tree, rosalina, and palmarosa can help to soothe inflammation and kill bad bacteria in the vagina.

ANTIBACTERIAL SITZ BATH

MAKES 1 TREATMENT ⤙ TOPICAL

1 cup witch hazel   ¼ cup aloe vera gel
5 drops lavender essential oil   1 cup sea salt
3 drops tea tree essential oil

1. In a medium bowl, stir together the witch hazel, lavender, and tea tree essential oils with the aloe vera gel.

2. Place the sea salt in another medium bowl and stir in the aloe vera mixture.

3. Pour the mixture under the running bath water, filling the tub quarter to half full.

4. Sit in the bath and soak the bottom half of your body for at least 20 minutes.

AWESOME ADDITION Soothing antibacterial herbs such as lavender and calendula make great additions to this sitz bath. Add ½ cup of each herb to a cloth tea bag or an old, clean sock, and tie closed before tossing into the bathtub.

ANTIBACTERIAL VAGINAL CLEANSING WIPES

MAKES 24 WIPES ⊱ TOPICAL

1 tablespoon unrefined coconut oil
5 drops lavender essential oil

3 drops tea tree essential oil
½ cup lavender hydrosol

1. In a small pan over low heat, melt the coconut oil. Add the lavender and tea tree essential oils, and stir to combine.

2. Place the lavender hydrosol in a small bowl then whisk in the coconut oil mixture.

3. Cut 12 paper towels in half and stack them in a glass container that has a lid. Pour the lavender mixture over the paper towel stack. The paper towels should soak up all the liquid.

4. Cover the wipes with the lid. When not using, store in the refrigerator for up to 1 month.

BACTERIA-FIGHTING TAMPON

MAKES 4 TAMPONS ⊱ TOPICAL

½ cup unrefined coconut oil
3 drops lavender essential oil

1 drop tea tree essential oil
4 organic tampons

1. In a small pan over low heat, melt the coconut oil.

2. Remove from heat and pour into a Mason jar. Add the lavender and tea tree essential oils and stir to combine.

3. Dip each of the tampons into the oil mixture until soaked through. Place into a zip-top bag and put into the freezer for 20 minutes to harden. Store in the refrigerator.

4. To use, insert a tampon into the vagina at bedtime every night for 7 nights in a row. Remove first thing in the morning. Repeat as necessary.

AWESOME ADDITION To make these tampons even more soothing and effective, you can first infuse the coconut oil with soothing antibacterial herbs including lavender, chamomile, rosemary, calendula, and plantain. Simply steep the oil and herbs over low heat for 2 hours, then strain before use.

Headaches

Headaches are commonly a symptom of other issues within the body. There are many reasons a headache might attack, including lack of sleep, lack of water or food, low blood sugar, hormones, vitamin deficiency, magnesium deficiency, caffeine detox, sugar detox, and even from artificial fragrances in the air. While essential oils can help to soothe a headache, it is best to look at the reason for the headache and treat it accordingly. Essential oils that can help soothe a headache include lavender, spearmint, ginger, chamomile, petitgrain, rosalina, helichrysum, black pepper, blue tansy, neroli, marjoram, fir needle, cypress, juniper berry, and frankincense.

SOOTHING HEADACHE ROLL-ON
MAKES ⅓ OUNCE ❧ TOPICAL ❧ AROMATIC

1 drop lavender essential oil
1 drop marjoram essential oil

1 drop rosalina essential oil
Fractionated coconut oil

1. Add the lavender, marjoram, and rosalina essential oils to a ⅓-ounce glass roll-on bottle, then fill the bottle with the fractionated coconut oil. Place the roller ball and cap on and gently swirl to combine. Label your remedy.
2. To use, roll onto the back of your neck and temples whenever you feel a headache coming on.

TENSION-RELIEVING BATH
MAKES 1 TREATMENT ❧ TOPICAL ❧ AROMATIC

3 drops lemon essential oil
2 drops cypress essential oil
2 drops lavender essential oil
1 drop Roman chamomile essential oil

1 tablespoon unscented
   shampoo or castile soap
1 cup Epsom salt

1. In a small bowl, stir together the lemon, cypress, lavender, and Roman chamomile essential oils with the shampoo or soap.
2. Place the Epsom salt in a medium bowl and stir in the soap mixture.
3. Pour the mixture under the running bath water as you fill the tub.

SUBSTITUTION TIP Instead of unscented soap, you can alternately use your favorite carrier oil in this recipe, but be cautious when exiting because the oil will make the tub very slippery.

HEADACHE RELIEVER AROMATHERAPY INHALER
MAKES 1 TREATMENT ≫ AROMATIC

10 drops lavender essential oil
8 drops fir needle essential oil

8 drops spearmint essential oil
4 drops Roman chamomile essential oil

1. Combine all the essential oils in a small glass bowl.
2. Using tweezers, add the wick (the cotton pad) of an aromatherapy personal inhaler to the bowl and roll it around until it's soaked up all of the essential oils mixture.
3. Use the tweezers to transfer the wick to the inhaler tube. Close the tube and label the inhaler.
4. Take a whiff of the inhaler whenever you feel a headache coming on.

Heartburn

Heartburn, the feeling of burning in the chest and/or throat, occurs when stomach acid rises up from the stomach into the esophagus. This annoyingly uncomfortable condition is completely normal during pregnancy and can increase the closer you get to your due date. There are many essential oils that can help soothe heartburn, including spearmint, ginger, lemon, sweet orange, tangerine, mandarin, grapefruit, chamomile, lavender, marjoram, coriander, cypress, and bergamot.

SOOTHE THE BURN AROMATHERAPY ROLL-ON
MAKES ⅓ OUNCE ≫ TOPICAL ≫ AROMATIC

2 drops tangerine essential oil
1 drop coriander essential oil

1 drop spearmint essential oil
Fractionated coconut oil

1. Add the tangerine, coriander, and spearmint essential oils to a ⅓-ounce glass roll-on bottle, then fill the bottle with the fractionated coconut oil. Place the roller ball and cap on, and gently swirl to combine. Label your creation. ➤

2. To use, roll onto your chest, wrists, and the back of your neck whenever you feel heartburn coming on.

SUBSTITUTION TIP If you don't have tangerine essential oil on hand, substitute sweet orange or mandarin essential oils. Tangerine and sweet orange essential oils have very similar scent profiles and can be interchanged freely in all recipes.

ANTACID AROMATHERAPY INHALER
MAKES 1 TREATMENT ❧ AROMATIC

15 drops lemon essential oil
10 drops ginger essential oil

5 drops Roman chamomile essential oil

1. Combine all the essential oils in a small glass bowl.
2. Using tweezers, add the wick (the cotton pad) of an aromatherapy personal inhaler to the bowl and roll it around until it's soaked up all of the essential oils mixture.
3. Use the tweezers to transfer the wick to the inhaler tube. Close the tube and label the inhaler.
4. Take a whiff of the inhaler whenever you have heartburn.

DIGESTIVE DIFFUSER BLEND
MAKES ½ OUNCE ❧ AROMATIC ❧ PHOTOSENSITIZING

1 teaspoon lemon essential oil
¾ teaspoon spearmint essential oil

¾ teaspoon sweet orange essential oil
½ teaspoon Roman chamomile essential oil

1. Add all the essential oils to an empty essential oil bottle (or any dark glass bottle with a dropper) and gently swirl the bottle to combine.
2. Add 10 drops to a diffuser and diffuse throughout the room in 10 to 15 minute increments (10 to 15 minutes on/30 minutes off) to avoid overexposure.

HELPFUL HINT Dilute this blend in coconut oil to rub on your chest and body. Because the blend contains lemon essential oil, which is photosensitizing, don't forget to dilute before using topically and to use caution in the sun.

Hemorrhoids

Hemorrhoids, or piles, are swollen veins in the rectum and anus. They can be a common occurrence during the last two trimesters of pregnancy because the baby is putting extra pressure on the blood vessels in the pelvis. Oftentimes, hemorrhoids can easily be treated with natural remedies, including herbs and essential oils. Antibacterial and anti-inflammatory essential oils such as lavender, tea tree, cypress, chamomile, geranium, frankincense, helichrysum, sandalwood, and juniper berry are all great at soothing and shrinking piles.

ANTIBACTERIAL HEMORRHOID CLEANSING WIPES
MAKES 24 WIPES ≫ TOPICAL

1 tablespoon unrefined coconut oil
5 drops lavender essential oil
3 drops cypress essential oil

¼ cup plus 2 tablespoons witch hazel
2 tablespoons aloe vera gel

1. In a small pan over low heat, melt the coconut oil. Add the lavender and cypress essential oils, and stir to combine.
2. Place the witch hazel into a small glass bowl. Whisk in the aloe vera gel and coconut oil mixture.
3. Cut 12 paper towels in half and stack them in a glass container that has a lid. Pour the mixture over the paper towel stack. The paper towels should soak up all the liquid.
4. Cover the wipes with the lid. When not using, store in the refrigerator for up to 1 month.

HEMORRHOID RELIEF SALVE
MAKES 4 OUNCES ≫ TOPICAL

¼ cup unrefined coconut oil
2 tablespoons beeswax
2 tablespoons unrefined shea butter

16 drops cypress essential oil
10 drops German chamomile essential oil
10 drops lavender essential oil

1. In a small pan over low heat, melt the coconut oil, beeswax, and shea butter. ➤

2. Once melted, remove from heat, add the cypress, German chamomile, and lavender essential oils, and stir to combine.

3. Pour into a Mason jar, and put into the freezer for 20 minutes to harden. Store in a cool, dark location.

4. To use, apply a dime-size amount of the salve to the affected areas.

HEALING HEMORRHOID SITZ BATH

MAKES 1 TREATMENT ❧ TOPICAL

1 cup witch hazel
5 drops lavender essential oil
3 drops geranium essential oil

¼ cup aloe vera gel
1 cup sea salt

1. In a small bowl, stir together the witch hazel, lavender, and geranium essential oils with the aloe vera gel.

2. Place the sea salt in a medium bowl and stir in the aloe vera mixture.

3. Pour the mixture under the running bath water, filling the tub quarter to half full.

4. Sit in the bath and soak the bottom half of your body for at least 20 minutes.

AWESOME ADDITION Soothing anti-inflammatory herbs such as lavender, plantain leaves, sage, or St. John's wort, all make great additions to this sitz bath. Add ½ cup of each herb you'd like to a cloth tea bag or an old, clean sock, and tie closed before tossing into the bathtub.

Insomnia

Everyone tells pregnant mamas to get as much sleep as possible before the baby comes, but it's easier said than done. There are many reasons that you might find yourself awake at night while pregnant, from the awkward belly size to the constant need to pee, but essential oils can help to calm the mind and relax the body so that you can get a good night's rest. The best essential oils for sleep include lavender, chamomile, marjoram, rosalina, sweet orange, tangerine, cedarwood, petitgrain, ylang-ylang, bergamot, coriander, frankincense, mandarin, vetiver, and sandalwood.

GOOD NIGHT SLEEP TIGHT AROMATHERAPY ROLL-ON

MAKES ⅓ OUNCE ❧ TOPICAL ❧ AROMATIC ❧ PHOTOSENSITIZING

1 drop bergamot essential oil
1 drop lavender essential oil
1 drop Roman chamomile essential oil

1 drop sweet orange essential oil
Fractionated coconut oil

1. Add the bergamot, lavender, Roman chamomile, and sweet orange essential oils to a ⅓-ounce glass roll-on bottle, then fill with the fractionated coconut oil. Place the roller ball and cap on, and gently swirl to combine. Label your creation.

2. To use, roll onto the back of your neck, chest, temples, and wrists before lying down to sleep.

SWEET DREAMS DIFFUSER BLEND

MAKES ½ OUNCE ❧ AROMATIC

1 teaspoon lavender essential oil
1 teaspoon marjoram essential oil

½ teaspoon Atlas cedarwood essential oil
½ teaspoon Roman chamomile essential oil

1. Add all of the essential oils to an empty essential oil bottle (or any dark glass bottle with a dropper), and gently swirl the bottle to combine.

2. Add 10 drops to a diffuser and diffuse throughout the room in 10 to 15 minute increments (10 to 15 minutes on/30 minutes off) to avoid overexposure.

HELPFUL HINT Dilute the blend in coconut oil to rub on your body, or even add to your favorite lotion for a moisturizing bedtime lotion. The blend is strong, so don't forget to dilute before using topically.

MOONLIGHT MAMA RELAXING BATH

MAKES 1 TREATMENT ❧ TOPICAL ❧ AROMATIC

5 drops lavender essential oil
3 drops sweet orange essential oil
2 drops neroli essential oil

1 tablespoon unscented
 shampoo or castile soap
1 cup Epsom salt

1. In a small bowl, stir together the lavender, sweet orange, and neroli essential oils with the shampoo or liquid soap. ➤

2. Place the Epsom salt in a medium bowl and stir in the soap mixture.

3. Pour the mixture under the running bath water as you fill the tub.

SUBSTITUTION TIP Instead of unscented soap, you can alternately use your favorite carrier oil, but be cautious when exiting because the oil will make the tub very slippery.

Leg Cramps

More than half of all pregnant women experience leg cramps and spasms during the second and third trimesters. Leg cramps can range from mild to severe and are more prominent at nighttime, when swelling is as its worst and fluid builds up. Anti-inflammatory and circulatory promoting essential oils such as lavender, marjoram, rosalina, helichrysum, cypress, petitgrain, juniper berry, lemon, frankincense, coriander, black pepper, and fir needle are the best to use when leg cramps strike.

ANTISPASMODIC MASSAGE OIL
MAKES 4 OUNCES ⊱ TOPICAL

½ cup unrefined coconut oil

16 drops lavender essential oil

10 drops helichrysum essential oil

10 drops marjoram essential oil

1. In a medium pot over low heat, melt the coconut oil.

2. Once melted, remove from heat, add the lavender, helichrysum, and marjoram essential oils, and stir to combine.

3. Pour into a Mason jar, and put into the freezer for 20 minutes to harden. Store in a cool, dark location.

4. To use, apply a small amount of oil to the cramping area and massage it in.

AWESOME ADDITION Arnica flowers and St. John's wort are herbs well known for their anti-inflammatory and nervine (nerve-soothing) properties and make a great addition to any pain relief oil. Steep 2 tablespoons arnica flowers and 2 tablespoons St. John's wort in the coconut oil over low heat for a couple of hours. Strain before using in this recipe.

LEMON ROSEMARY ANTI-INFLAMMATORY BATH
MAKES 1 TREATMENT

5 drops lavender essential oil
3 drops cypress essential oil
3 drops lemon essential oil

1 tablespoon unscented
   shampoo or castile soap
1 cup Epsom salt

1. In a small bowl, stir together the lavender, cypress, and lemon essential oils with the liquid soap to combine.
2. Place the Epsom salt in a medium bowl and stir in the soap mixture.
3. Pour the salt mixture under the running bath water as you fill the tub.

AWESOME ADDITION Rosemary and lavender are pain relieving herbs that can help improve circulation and relieve muscles and nerve pains. Add ½ cup of each herb to a cloth tea bag or an old, clean sock, and tie closed before tossing into the bathtub.

Morning Sickness

More than 50 percent of pregnant women experience morning sickness during pregnancy. Essential oils can be very helpful in relieving the symptoms of nausea. Simply inhaling essential oils of ginger, citrus, or spearmint can help calm nausea and soothe an upset stomach. In rare cases, morning sickness is so severe that it can require hospitalization, anti-nausea medications, and even IV fluids. Morning sickness this severe is called *hyperemesis gravidarum*. Contact your medical practitioner if you experience severe nausea and vomiting that won't quit, can't keep any fluids down, have dark-colored urine, or are fainting and/or vomiting blood.

ANTI-NAUSEA AROMATHERAPY INHALER
MAKES 1 TREATMENT ✻ AROMATIC

10 drops ginger essential oil
10 drops lemon essential oil

10 drops sweet orange essential oil

1. Combine all the essential oils in a small glass bowl.
2. Using tweezers, add the wick (the cotton pad) of an aromatherapy personal inhaler to the bowl and roll it around until it's soaked up all of the essential oils mixture. ➔

3. Use the tweezers to transfer the wick to the inhaler tube. Close the tube and label the inhaler.

4. Take a whiff of the inhaler whenever you feel nauseated.

MORNING SICKNESS DIFFUSER BLEND
MAKES ½ OUNCE ➤ AROMATIC ➤ PHOTOSENSITIZING

1¼ teaspoons sweet orange essential oil   ¾ teaspoon spearmint essential oil
1 teaspoon grapefruit essential oil

1. Add all the essential oils to a 5-ml bottle, and gently swirl the bottle to combine.

2. Add 10 drops to a diffuser and diffuse throughout the room in 10 to 15 minute increments (10 to 15 minutes on/30 minutes off) to prevent overexposure.

HELPFUL HINT Dilute this blend in coconut oil to rub on your chest and body, or add it to your favorite lotion. This blend contains photosensitizing grapefruit oil, so don't forget to dilute it before using topically, and use caution in the sun.

Pre-eclampsia

Pre-eclampsia is a rare but dangerous condition, requiring immediate medical attention. It usually occurs during the third trimester and causes high blood pressure, abnormally high protein in urine, and water retention. If left untreated, it can lead to organ damage and seizures. Symptoms include headaches, nausea, dizziness, and swollen ankles. Consult your doctor if you suspect pre-eclampsia. The following remedies are great preventive aids or can be used in conjunction with medical treatment. **They do *not* replace medical attention or your doctor's advice.** Essential oils that help to calm the mind and body, such as lavender, chamomile, rosalina, bergamot, sweet orange, coriander, marjoram, ylang-ylang, frankincense, mandarin, tangerine, cedarwood, sandalwood, petitgrain, vetiver, vanilla, and blue tansy are perfect oils to use with medical treatment.

STRESS-RELIEVING DIFFUSER BLEND

MAKES ½ OUNCE ❧ AROMATIC ❧ PHOTOSENSITIZING

1 teaspoon lavender essential oil

1 teaspoon bergamot essential oil

½ teaspoon Roman chamomile essential oil

½ teaspoon frankincense essential oil

1. Add all the essential oils to an empty essential oil bottle (or any dark glass bottle with a dropper), and gently swirl the bottle to combine.
2. Add 10 drops to a diffuser and diffuse throughout the room in 10 to 15 minute increments (10 to 15 minutes on/30 minutes off) to avoid overexposure.

HELPFUL HINT Dilute the blend in coconut oil or your favorite unscented lotion and massage all over your body. This blend contains phototoxic bergamot oil, so don't forget to dilute before using topically, and use caution before going out in the sun.

CHILLAXIN' MASSAGE OIL

MAKES 4 OUNCES ❧ TOPICAL

½ cup unrefined coconut oil or similar carrier oil

16 drops rosalina essential oil

10 drops coriander essential oil

10 drops lavender essential oil

1. In a small pan over low heat, melt the coconut oil.
2. Once melted, remove from heat, add the essential oils, and stir to combine.
3. Pour into a Mason jar and store in a cool, dark location.
4. Have your partner gently massage you with this oil wherever you feel comfortable. Relax and breathe.

MEDITATING MAMA ROOM SPRAY

MAKES 6 OUNCES ❧ AROMATIC

25 drops sweet orange essential oil
15 drops lavender essential oil
10 drops frankincense essential oil

2 tablespoons 80-proof vodka
5 ounces filtered water

1. Add all the ingredients to a spray bottle and shake to combine.
2. Spray around the room and on pillows and furniture to enjoy the scent throughout the room. Remember to breathe in, too.

SUBSTITUTION TIP Witch hazel makes a great substitute for vodka in a room spray. Be sure to shake the bottle well before spraying, though. Witch hazel contains only a small percentage of alcohol and the essential oils will not mix like they would with the vodka.

Pregnancy Fatigue

Most women experience fatigue during pregnancy, especially during the first trimester. Fatigue happens for many reasons including hormone fluctuations, dehydration, anemia, low blood pressure, low blood sugar, and even poor nutrition. Be sure to drink plenty of water and eat small snacks throughout the day. When you need a refreshing breath, essential oils are a great way to energize and wake you up. Spearmint, lemon, grapefruit, ginger, lemon eucalyptus, cypress, pine, fir needle, geranium, and coriander essential oils all help to keep you going when your energy is waning.

WAKE UP AND GO-GO AROMATHERAPY INHALER

MAKES 1 TREATMENT ❧ AROMATIC

10 drops grapefruit essential oil
10 drops lemon essential oil

5 drops coriander essential oil
5 drops spearmint essential oil

1. Combine all the essential oils in a small glass bowl.
2. Using tweezers, add the wick (the cotton pad) of an aromatherapy personal inhaler to the bowl and roll it around until it's soaked up all of the essential oils mixture.

3. Use the tweezers to transfer the wick to the inhaler tube. Close the tube and label the inhaler.

4. Take a whiff of the inhaler whenever you need an energy boost.

GET UP AND GO DIFFUSER BLEND
MAKES ½ OUNCE ≫ AROMATIC ≫ PHOTOSENSITIZING

1 teaspoon grapefruit essential oil
¾ teaspoon ginger essential oil

¾ teaspoon lemon eucalyptus essential oil
½ teaspoon fir needle essential oil

1. Add all the essential oils to an empty essential oil bottle (or any dark glass bottle with a dropper), and gently swirl the bottle to combine.

2. Add 10 drops to a diffuser and diffuse throughout the room in 10 to 15 minute increments (10 to 15 minutes on/30 minutes off) to avoid overexposure.

HELPFUL HINT This blend contains photosensitizing grapefruit oil, so don't forget to dilute it before using topically, and use caution before going out in the sun.

GO, GO, GO AROMATHERAPY ROLL-ON
MAKES ⅓ OUNCE ≫ TOPICAL ≫ AROMATIC

1 drop bergamot essential oil
1 drop coriander essential oil

1 drop cypress essential oil
Fractionated coconut oil

1. Add the bergamot, coriander, and cypress essential oils to a ⅓-ounce glass roll-on bottle, then add fractionated coconut oil to fill. Place the roller ball and cap on, and gently swirl to combine. Label your creation.

2. To use, roll onto the back of your neck, chest, and wrists whenever you need an energy boost.

SUBSTITUTION TIP Cypress, pine, and fir needle essential oils can usually be interchanged freely in most recipes.

PUPPP (Pruritic Urticarial Papules and Plaques of Pregnancy)

As the belly begins to grow and the skin stretches, some women develop PUPPP, itching and rashes that are associated with an allergic reaction to the skin stretching—although there is still not enough evidence to prove this hypothesis, and the condition is not completely understood. Natural remedies, including topical application of soothing anti-inflammatory essential oils such as lavender, chamomile, geranium, blue tansy, rosalina, sandalwood, helichrysum, patchouli, and spearmint, are very helpful at reducing itching, calming the rash, and healing the skin.

SOOTHING ANTI-ITCH PASTE
MAKES 3 OUNCES ❧ TOPICAL

¼ cup bentonite clay
2 tablespoons baking soda
1 tablespoon vegetable glycerin
1 tablespoon aloe vera gel

10 drops lavender essential oil
5 drops rosalina essential oil
5 drops spearmint essential oil
Witch hazel

1. In a small glass bowl, combine the bentonite clay and baking soda.
2. Mix in the vegetable glycerin, aloe vera gel, and lavender, rosalina, and spearmint essential oils. Add enough witch hazel to form a paste. Store in the refrigerator when not using.
3. To use, apply to itchy skin and rashes as often as needed.

SUBSTITUTION TIP You can substitute peppermint hydrosol for witch hazel since it is known for soothing and healing itchy skin and rashes. You might also try this recipe with lavender or calendula hydrosol.

ITCH-B-GONE OAT BATH
MAKES 1 TREATMENT → TOPICAL

1 cup oats

¼ cup baking soda

10 drops lavender essential oil

5 drops blue tansy essential oil

1. Pulse oats in a blender or food processor until powdered. Add the baking soda and pulse until everything is well mixed.
2. Add the lavender and blue tansy essential oils, and pulse a few times more to mix in.
3. To use, add straight to the bath under running water, or place in a fine mesh bag or an old, clean sock, tie closed, and toss into the bathtub under the running water. Soak in the tub at least 20 minutes. Store any unused treatment in a Mason jar in a cool, dry location.

HELPFUL HINT To keep skin moisturized, do not wipe dry after getting out of the tub. Gently pat your skin dry instead and immediately apply a healing body butter or Soothe the Itch Salve (below).

SOOTHE THE ITCH SALVE
MAKES 4 OUNCES → TOPICAL

¼ cup extra-virgin olive oil

2 tablespoons beeswax

2 tablespoons unrefined shea butter

16 drops rosalina essential oil

10 drops German chamomile essential oil

10 drops lavender essential oil

1. In a small pan over low heat, melt the olive oil, beeswax, and shea butter.
2. Once melted, remove from heat and add the rosalina, chamomile, and lavender essential oils.
3. Pour into a Mason jar and put into the freezer for 20 minutes to harden. (Store any unused salve in a cool, dark location.)
4. To use, apply the salve to itchy skin and rashes whenever needed.

AWESOME ADDITION Activated charcoal is naturally able to soothe itching and rashes. Add 1 tablespoon to this recipe, then stir well to combine. The charcoal will change the color of this salve to black, so be cautious when applying around light clothing.

Round Ligament Pains

Round ligament pains—the stretching of the circular ligament in the pelvic region—is caused by hormonal changes and your growing baby bump, creating sharp pains in the pelvic region under the bump. Maternity belts, yoga stretches, and walking all help alleviate some of the pain. Massages using anti-inflammatory and pain relieving essential oils, including lavender, chamomile, rosalina, black pepper, petitgrain, ginger, marjoram, helichrysum, sandalwood, frankincense, cypress, fir needle, ylang-ylang, patchouli, blue tansy, spearmint, geranium, and juniper berry, can also help.

ROUND LIGAMENT MASSAGE OIL #1
MAKES 4 OUNCES ⤳ TOPICAL

½ cup extra-virgin olive oil
16 drops ginger essential oil

10 drops black pepper essential oil
10 drops lavender essential oil

1. Combine the olive oil with the ginger, black pepper, and lavender essential oils in a bottle. (Store any unused oil in a cool, dark location.)
2. To use, apply a small amount to the area that aches, and massage in.

AWESOME ADDITION St. John's wort-infused oil is a common remedy for muscle and nerve pains alike. Infuse ¼ cup St. John's wort into the olive oil over low heat for 2 hours. Strain the herbs from the oil before using in this recipe.

ROUND LIGAMENT MASSAGE OIL #2
MAKES 4 OUNCES ⤳ TOPICAL

½ cup unrefined coconut oil
16 drops marjoram essential oil

10 drops black pepper essential oil
10 drops helichrysum essential oil

1. In a small pan over low heat, melt the coconut oil.
2. Once melted, remove from heat, add the marjoram, black pepper, and helichrysum essential oils, and stir to combine.
3. Pour into a Mason jar, and put into the freezer for 20 minutes to harden. (Store any unused oil in a cool, dark location.)
4. Apply a small amount to the area that aches and massage in.

Sciatica

Sciatic nerve pain, usually caused in pregnancy by pressure on the sciatic nerve from water retention or weight gain, includes symptoms such as weakness, numbness, tingling, and/or shooting pains in the legs. Yoga and essential oil massages can help relieve some of the nerve pains. Helpful antispasmodic and anti-inflammatory essential oils include lavender, rosalina, spearmint, petitgrain, marjoram, black pepper, turmeric CO_2, cypress, fir needle, juniper berry, frankincense, helichrysum, geranium, sandalwood, ginger, tangerine, patchouli, blue tansy, and ylang-ylang.

SCIATIC RELIEF MASSAGE OIL #1
MAKES 4 OUNCES ❧ TOPICAL

½ cup unrefined coconut oil

16 drops marjoram essential oil

10 drops cypress essential oil

10 drops helichrysum essential oil

1. In a small pan over low heat, melt the coconut oil.
2. Once melted, remove from heat, add the marjoram, cypress, and helichrysum essential oils, and stir to combine.
3. Pour into a Mason jar, and put into the freezer for 20 minutes to harden. Store any unused oil in a cool, dark location.
4. To use, apply a small amount to the area that aches and massage in.

SCIATIC RELIEF MASSAGE OIL #2
MAKES 4 OUNCES ❧ TOPICAL

½ cup extra-virgin olive oil

16 drops lavender essential oil

10 drops ginger essential oil

10 drops turmeric CO_2

1. Combine the olive oil and the lavender, ginger, and turmeric essential oils in a bottle. (Store any unused oil in a cool, dark location.)
2. To use, apply a small amount to the area that aches and massage the oil in.

AWESOME ADDITION St. John's wort-infused oil is a common remedy for muscle and nerve pains alike. Infuse ¼ cup St. John's wort into the olive oil over low heat for 2 hours. Strain the herbs from the oil before using in this recipe.

SOOTHE YOUR NERVES HERBAL BATH
MAKES 1 TREATMENT ❧ TOPICAL ❧ AROMATIC

5 drops lavender essential oil
3 drops marjoram essential oil
2 drops sandalwood essential oil

1 tablespoon unscented
   shampoo or castile soap
1 cup Epsom salt

1. In a small bowl, stir together the lavender, marjoram, and sandalwood essential oils with the shampoo or liquid soap.

2. Place the Epsom salt in a medium bowl and stir in the soap mixture.

3. Pour the mixture under the running bath water as you fill the tub.

AWESOME ADDITION Soothing antispasmodic herbs such as lavender and St. John's wort make great additions to this bath. Add ¼ cup of each herb to a cloth tea bag or an old, clean sock, and tie closed before tossing into the bathtub.

Stretch Marks

I got very lucky during my pregnancy and managed to make it through without a single stretch mark to show for it. My secret was applying my homemade body butter all over my body every day. While there are no guarantees that a daily routine of massaging a balm or butter all over your belly will prevent you from gaining stretch marks, you are probably far more likely to end up with stretch marks if you don't. Using butters, oils, and lotions daily during your pregnancy helps keep your skin moisturized and more capable of stretching without leaving marks behind. Many oils and butters contain vitamins A, C, and E, as well as other scar-minimizing benefits.

STRETCH MARK MASSAGE OIL
MAKES ABOUT 4 OUNCES ❧ TOPICAL

¼ cup avocado oil
20 drops lavender essential oil
5 drops frankincense essential oil
5 drops geranium essential oil

2 tablespoons rosehip seed oil
2 tablespoons tamanu oil
1 teaspoon vitamin E oil

1. Combine all the ingredients in a bottle, and gently swirl to combine.

2. Massage the oil onto your belly, back, butt, and thighs twice a day.

MAMA'S BELLY BUTTER

MAKES 8 OUNCES ☙ TOPICAL

½ cup unrefined mango butter
¼ cup unrefined coconut oil
¼ cup rosehip seed oil

40 drops steam-distilled lemon
 essential oil (see Tip)
20 drops neroli essential oil
1 teaspoon vitamin E oil

1. In a small pan over low heat, melt the mango butter and coconut oil.

2. Once melted, remove from heat and add the rosehip seed oil, the steam-distilled lemon and neroli essential oils, and vitamin E oil.

3. Pour the mixture into an 8-ounce Mason jar, and put into the freezer for 20 minutes to harden. Alternately, you can whip the butter using a hand mixer or emulsion blender for 3 to 5 minutes, after hardening most of the way. Don't let it get fully hardened so that it's easier to whip into a light fluffy texture. If you whipped too soon and it's still not solid enough, simply place in the freezer for a tiny bit longer before whipping again.

4. To use, apply twice a day throughout your pregnancy and twice a day postpartum, as your belly shrinks back down, to prevent scarring.

SAFETY TIP Steam-distilled, instead of cold-pressed, lemon essential oil makes this belly butter safe to wear, even when you are having fun out in the sun! You can substitute photosensitizing cold-pressed lemon essential oil, but be sure not to apply the belly butter before exposing your belly to sunlight. If you will be covering the skin or staying indoors, cold-pressed lemon essential oil is completely safe.

Urinary Tract Infections

Urinary tract infections (UTIs) are common for many women during pregnancy. You know you have a UTI when you notice the telltale signs of burning while urinating, the constant urge to pee even when you have none left, and cloudy, strong-smelling pee. Drinking cranberry juice is one of the best natural treatments and preventions of UTIs. Essential oils can be used in soothing baths and wipes to cleanse, soothe, and treat the UTI. Antibacterial and anti-inflammatory essential oils such as lavender, rosalina, tea tree, blue tansy, chamomile, geranium, helichrysum, sweet orange, and neroli can help reduce pain and inflammation while healing up the infection.

SOOTHING HERBAL SITZ BATH

MAKES 1 TREATMENT ❧ TOPICAL

5 drops lavender essential oil
5 drops rosalina essential oil
1 tablespoon aloe vera gel

1 cup Epsom salt
1 cup raw unfiltered apple
  cider vinegar

1. In a small bowl, stir together the lavender and rosalina essential oils with the aloe vera gel.

2. Place the Epsom salt in a medium bowl and stir in the aloe vera mixture and apple cider vinegar.

3. Pour the mixture under the running bath water, filling the tub only a quarter to half full.

4. Sit in the bath and soak the bottom half of your body for at least 20 minutes.

AWESOME ADDITION Soothing antibacterial herbs such as lavender and calendula make great additions to this sitz bath. Add ¼ cup of each herb to a cloth tea bag or an old, clean sock, and tie closed before tossing into the bathtub.

CLEANSING ANTIBACTERIAL WIPES

MAKES 24 WIPES ❧ TOPICAL

1 tablespoon unrefined coconut oil
5 drops lavender essential oil
5 drops tea tree essential oil

¼ cup plus 2 tablespoons witch hazel
2 tablespoons aloe vera gel

1. In a small pan over low heat, melt the coconut oil. Add the lavender and tea tree essential oils and stir to combine.

2. Place the witch hazel and aloe vera gel into a small glass bowl. Whisk the coconut oil mixture into the witch hazel mixture.

3. Cut 12 paper towels in half and stack them in a glass container that has a lid. Pour over the stack of paper towels. The paper towels should soak up all the liquid.

4. Cover the wipes with the lid. Store in the refrigerator when not using, for up to 1 month.

Varicose Veins

Varicose veins are pesky twisted veins that are larger than normal and sit at the surface of the skin, where you can see them. They are usually found in the legs, ankles, and all the way up the thighs to the vagina. Like hemorrhoids, they can be very painful and require gentle anti-inflammatory compression rather than massages. Soothing anti-inflammatory and circulatory promoting essential oils such as lavender, rosalina, cedarwood, geranium, ginger, lemon, neroli, cypress, chamomile, blue tansy, fir needle, frankincense, helichrysum, sandalwood, grapefruit, and juniper berry are all great at soothing and shrinking varicose veins.

VARICOSE VEINS SITZ BATH

MAKES 1 TREATMENT ≫ TOPICAL

5 drops cypress essential oil
3 drops lavender essential oil
2 drops blue tansy essential oil

1 tablespoon aloe vera gel
1 cup Epsom salt
1 cup witch hazel

1. In a medium bowl, stir together the cypress, lavender, and blue tansy essential oils with the aloe vera gel.
2. Place the Epsom salt in another medium bowl and stir in the aloe vera mixture.
3. Pour the mixture and the witch hazel under the running bath water, filling the tub quarter to half full.
4. Sit in the bath and soak the bottom half of your body for at least 20 minutes.

AWESOME ADDITION Soothing anti-inflammatory herbs such as lavender and calendula make great additions to this sitz bath. Add ½ cup of each herb to a cloth tea bag or an old, clean sock, and tie it closed before tossing it into the bathtub.

VARICOSE VEINS SALVE

MAKES 4 OUNCES ❧ TOPICAL

¼ cup plus 2 tablespoons
  extra-virgin olive oil
2 tablespoons beeswax pastilles

16 drops Virginia cedarwood essential oil
10 drops lavender essential oil
10 drops lemon essential oil

1. In a small pan over low heat, melt the olive oil and beeswax.

2. Once melted, remove from heat, and add the Virginia cedarwood, lavender, and lemon essential oils.

3. Pour into a Mason jar, and put into the freezer for 20 minutes to harden. (Store any unused salve in a cool, dark location.)

4. To use, gently apply the salve to varicose veins. Do not massage or put pressure onto the veins.

GRAPEFRUIT-COFFEE VARICOSE VEIN OIL

MAKES 8 OUNCES ❧ TOPICAL ❧ PHOTOSENSITIZING

1 cup extra-virgin olive oil
½ cup ground coffee
30 drops grapefruit essential oil

20 drops lavender essential oil
15 drops helichrysum essential oil

1. In a small pan over low heat, steep the olive oil and coffee for 1 to 3 hours.

2. Using a fine mesh strainer or coffee filter, strain the oil.

3. Combine the grapefruit, lavender, and helichrysum essential oils with the coffee-infused olive oil in a bottle. (Store any unused oil in a cool, dark location.)

4. To use, very gently apply the oil to varicose veins. Do not massage or put pressure onto the veins.

HELPFUL HINT Compression socks work very well to help promote circulation and reduce inflammation. They can be worn after applying either the varicose veins salve or the grapefruit-coffee oil. Covering the skin after a topical application of essential oils helps them to work more effectively. Grapefruit oil causes photosensitization, so use caution when using this oil on any part of your body that might see the sun.

Yeast Infections

It's very common for women to get vaginal yeast infections during pregnancy. Caused by the growth of the fungus *Candida albicans*, vaginal yeast infections cause inflammation, intense itching, and a thick white discharge from the vagina. Yeast infections can be treated naturally by avoiding candida triggers such as sugar in your diet, the use of antibiotics, and proper cleanliness in the affected areas. Soothing antifungal essential oils including lavender, tea tree, coriander, sweet orange, lemon, mandarin, grapefruit, tangerine, geranium, chamomile, cedarwood, and frankincense can also help combat yeast infections.

ANTIFUNGAL VAGINAL WIPES

MAKES 24 WIPES ≫ TOPICAL

1 tablespoon unrefined coconut oil
5 drops lavender essential oil

5 drops tea tree essential oil
½ cup witch hazel

1. In a small pan over low heat, melt the coconut oil. Add the lavender and tea tree essential oils and stir to combine.
2. Place the witch hazel into a small glass bowl. Whisk the coconut oil mixture into the witch hazel
3. Cut 12 paper towels in half and stack them in a glass container that has a lid. Pour the mixture over the paper towel stack. The paper towels should soak up all the liquid.
4. Cover the wipes with the lid and store in the refrigerator when not using for up to 1 month.

YEASTY YONI POWDER

MAKES ½ CUP ≫ TOPICAL

½ cup acidophilus powder
5 drops geranium essential oil

5 drops lavender essential oil

1. Combine all the ingredients in a glass bowl. Stir until the essential oils are evenly distributed throughout the powder.
2. To use, sprinkle the powder onto your underwear or dust your vaginal area with it.

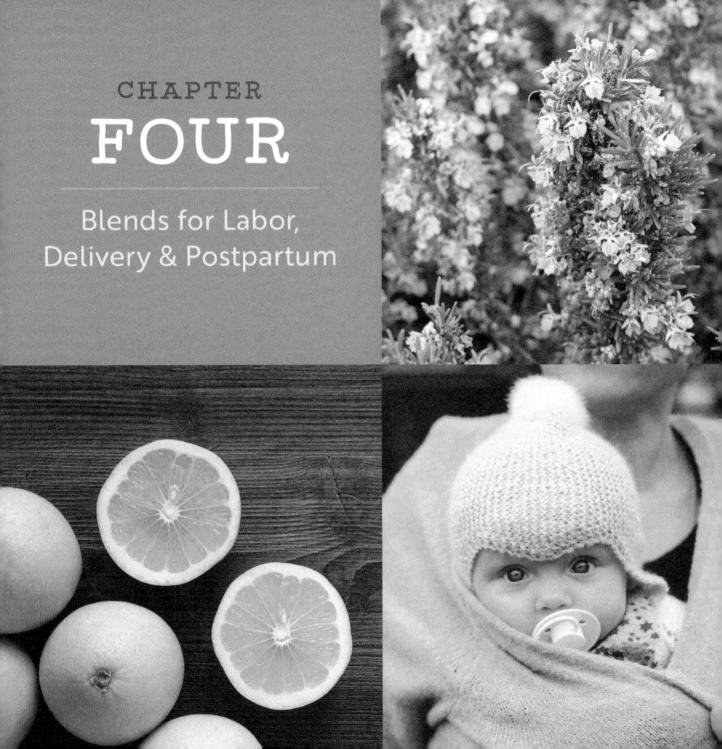

CHAPTER

FOUR

Blends for Labor, Delivery & Postpartum

Anxiety

Anxiety during labor and delivery is completely natural. Aromatherapy in the delivery room can help to calm fears and relieve stress. Stress- and anxiety-alleviating essential oils include lavender, chamomile, clary sage, lemon, sweet orange, grapefruit, petitgrain, coriander, bergamot, vanilla, sandalwood, ylang-ylang, cedarwood, and neroli.

CALM YOUR NERVES LABOR DIFFUSER BLEND
MAKES ½ OUNCE ❧ AROMATIC ❧ PHOTOSENSITIZING

1 teaspoon grapefruit essential oil
1 teaspoon lavender essential oil

½ teaspoon clary sage essential oil
½ teaspoon Roman chamomile essential oil

1. Add all the essential oils to an empty essential oil bottle (or any dark glass bottle with a dropper), and gently swirl the bottle to combine.
2. Add 10 drops to a diffuser and diffuse throughout the room in 30-minute increments (30 minutes on/30 minutes off) to avoid overexposure.

HELPFUL HINT Dilute the blend in coconut oil or your favorite unscented lotion and massage onto your body. This blend contains photosensitizing grapefruit oil, so don't forget to dilute before using topically, and use caution in the sun.

ANTI-ANXIETY AROMATHERAPY INHALER
MAKES 1 TREATMENT ❧ AROMATIC

10 drops grapefruit essential oil
10 drops sweet orange essential oil

5 drops clary sage essential oil
5 drops rosalina essential oil

1. Combine all the essential oils in a small glass bowl.
2. Using tweezers, add the wick (the cotton pad) of an aromatherapy personal inhaler to the bowl and roll it around until it's soaked up all of the essential oils mixture.
3. Use the tweezers to transfer the wick to the inhaler tube. Close the tube and label the inhaler.
4. Take a whiff of the inhaler whenever you need to relax and calm your mind.

CALM YOUR FEARS ROOM SPRAY

MAKES 6 OUNCES ✒ AROMATIC

5 ounces filtered water

2 tablespoons 80-proof vodka

20 drops lavender essential oil

10 drops frankincense essential oil

10 drops Roman chamomile essential oil

10 drops vanilla CO_2 (12%)

1. Add all the ingredients to a spray bottle and shake to combine.

2. Spray around the room and on pillows and furniture to enjoy the scent throughout the room.

SUBSTITUTION TIP If you don't have vodka on hand, witch hazel makes a great substitute in a room spray. Be sure to shake the bottle well before spraying. Witch hazel contains only a small percentage of alcohol and the essential oils will not mix into the water like they would with vodka.

After Pains

After giving birth, you might experience after pains (uterine cramping) as your uterus begins to contract back to its original size. These cramps are usually mild for first-time moms but can become more intense with each subsequent pregnancy. Essential oils with natural pain-relieving and anti-inflammatory properties such as lavender, chamomile, jasmine, geranium, rosalina, clary sage, marjoram, frankincense, cypress, fir needle, helichrysum, coriander, black pepper, petitgrain, bergamot, tangerine, balsam fir, ginger, lemon, and spruce can greatly reduce the occurrence of after pains. Jasmine absolute is a favorite because of its ability to promote uterine contractions and also provide pain relief.

SOOTHE YOUR AFTER PAINS HOT COMPRESS

MAKES 1 TREATMENT ✒ TOPICAL

2 tablespoons aloe vera gel

5 drops jasmine absolute

5 drops lavender essential oil

Boiling water

1. Add the aloe vera gel to a small bowl, then stir in the jasmine absolute and lavender essential oils.

2. Pour the water into a medium bowl and stir in the aloe vera mixture. →

3. To use, dip a washcloth into the mixture, squeeze out until damp. Apply to the abdomen.

AWESOME ADDITION Soothing anti-inflammatory herbs such as St. John's wort make great additions to this compress. Add ½ cup of the herb to a cloth tea bag or an old, clean sock, and tie closed before placing into the bowl of boiling water. Steep for 15 to 20 minutes before adding the mixture of aloe vera, jasmine, and lavender.

ANTISPASMODIC PAIN-RELIEVING SALVE
MAKES 4 OUNCES ⤳ TOPICAL

¼ cup plus 2 tablespoons
  extra-virgin olive oil
2 tablespoons beeswax pastilles

32 drops sweet marjoram essential oil
20 drops clary sage essential oil
20 drops frankincense essential oil

1. In a small pan over low heat, heat the olive oil and beeswax.
2. Once the beeswax is melted, remove from heat, and add the sweet marjoram, clary sage, and frankincense essential oils.
3. Pour into a Mason jar, and put into the freezer for 20 minutes to harden. (Store any unused salve in a cool, dark location.)
4. Apply the salve to the abdomen and lower back whenever needed.

Back Labor

Back labor occurs when the baby is not positioned correctly (head down toward pelvis, facing the spine) during labor, causing the mother intense pain in her lower back region. Thankfully, back labor can be managed with natural remedies, including essential oils and herbs. Pain-relieving and anti-inflammatory essential oils such as lavender, chamomile, rosalina, marjoram, frankincense, cypress, fir needle, helichrysum, coriander, black pepper, petitgrain, bergamot, tangerine, balsam fir, ginger, lemon, and spruce can help to relieve the pain.

PAIN-RELIEVING BACK LABOR MASSAGE OIL
MAKES 4 OUNCES ⤳ TOPICAL

½ cup unrefined coconut oil
32 drops lavender essential oil

20 drops rosalina essential oil
20 drops spearmint essential oil

1. In a small pan over low heat, melt the coconut oil.
2. Once melted, remove from heat, add the lavender, rosalina, and spearmint essential oils, and stir to combine.
3. Pour into a Mason jar, and put into the freezer for 20 minutes to harden. (Store any unused oil in a cool, dark location.)
4. To use, apply a small amount to the area that aches and massage in.

PUT YOUR BACK INTO IT SALVE
MAKES 4 OUNCES ➢ TOPICAL

¼ cup plus 2 tablespoons extra-virgin olive oil

2 tablespoons beeswax pastilles

32 drops marjoram essential oil

20 drops geranium essential oil

20 drops lavender essential oil

1. In a small pan over low heat, heat the olive oil and beeswax.
2. Once the beeswax is melted, remove from heat, and add the marjoram, geranium, and lavender essential oils.
3. Pour into a Mason jar, and put into the freezer for 20 minutes to harden. (Store the salve in a cool, dark location.)
4. To use, apply and massage into your lower back whenever pain occurs.

AWESOME ADDITION St. John's wort and arnica flowers both make great pain-relieving additions to this salve. Simply steep the olive oil with 2 tablespoons of each herb over low heat for 2 hours. Strain and then continue with the recipe.

BACK PAIN-RELIEVING LINIMENT SPRAY
MAKES 8 OUNCES ➢ TOPICAL

1 cup 80-proof vodka

¼ cup arnica flowers

¼ cup freshly minced ginger

10 drops lavender essential oil

5 drops marjoram essential oil

5 drops rosalina essential oil

1. Combine all the ingredients in a Mason jar. Cover and steep on the kitchen counter for 2 weeks. Shake the jar to mix the contents twice a day.
2. Strain the mixture into a spray bottle.
3. To use, spray onto your lower back and allow it to sink in.

Back Pains

It is normal for mamas to experience all sorts of aches and pains in the weeks that follow giving birth. Postpartum back pains are no exception. As your body changed to fit a baby in the womb, muscles in your back and abdomen were weakened and stretched during pregnancy and labor. As you build up the muscles needed to return to normal, essential oils can assist with managing the pain. Pain-relieving and anti-inflammatory essential oils such as lavender, chamomile, rosalina, marjoram, frankincense, cypress, petitgrain, fir needle, helichrysum, coriander, black pepper, bergamot, tangerine, balsam fir, ginger, lemon, turmeric CO_2, and spruce are great for this.

MUSCLE MENDER SALVE
MAKES 4 OUNCES ⇾ TOPICAL

¼ cup plus 2 tablespoons unrefined coconut oil
2 tablespoons beeswax pastilles
20 drops clary sage essential oil

20 drops lavender essential oil
20 drops marjoram essential oil
10 drops Roman chamomile essential oil

1. In a small pan over low heat, melt the coconut oil and beeswax.
2. Once melted, remove from heat, and add the clary sage, lavender, marjoram and Roman chamomile essential oils.
3. Pour into a Mason jar, and put into the freezer for 20 minutes to harden. (Store any unused salve in a cool, dark location.)
4. Apply the salve whenever needed.

AWESOME ADDITION Arnica flowers and St. John's wort are herbs well known for their anti-inflammatory and nervine properties and make a great addition to any pain relief oil or salve. Steep 2 tablespoons each of arnica flowers and St. John's wort in the coconut oil over low heat for 2 hours. Strain and continue with the recipe.

BACK BENDER LINIMENT

MAKES 8 OUNCES ❧ TOPICAL

1 cup 80-proof vodka
¼ cup arnica flowers
¼ cup St. John's wort

10 drops lavender essential oil
5 drops turmeric CO_2
4 drops rosalina essential oil

1. Combine all the ingredients in a Mason jar. Cover and steep on the kitchen counter for 2 weeks. Shake the jar to mix the contents twice a day.

2. Strain the mixture into a spray bottle.

3. To use, spray onto your back and allow it to sink in.

SUBSTITUTION TIP Witch hazel or vinegar can be substituted for the vodka in this recipe. Be sure to shake the bottle well before spraying. Witch hazel contains only a small percentage of alcohol and the essential oils will not mix into the witch hazel like they would with vodka.

Blocked Ducts and Mastitis

A blocked duct is a small swollen mass in the breast that is very painful. It is usually caused by infrequent breastfeeding. Blocked ducts typically cause the skin over the duct to turn red and if left untreated can lead to mastitis (inflammation of the mammary gland). The best way to clear a blocked duct is to breastfeed your baby often. Anti-inflammatory essential oils that help soothe the pain and inflammation, and promote healthy circulation for a blocked duct and mastitis include lavender, chamomile, rosalina, marjoram, frankincense, cypress, fir needle, helichrysum, coriander, black pepper, bergamot, tangerine, balsam fir, ginger, neroli, lemon, and spruce.

BLOCKED DUCT BOOBIE BALM

MAKES 4 OUNCES ❧ TOPICAL

¼ cup unrefined coconut oil

2 tablespoons beeswax pastilles

2 tablespoons unrefined shea butter

30 drops lavender essential oil

25 drops cypress essential oil

20 drops German chamomile essential oil

1. In a small pan over low heat, melt the coconut oil, beeswax, and shea butter.
2. Once melted, remove from heat and add the lavender, cypress, and German chamomile essential oils.
3. Pour into a Mason jar, and put into the freezer for 20 minutes to harden. (Store any unused balm in a cool, dark location.)
4. To use, apply the salve to affected areas directly after breastfeeding. Follow with a heated rice pack to the breast.

AWESOME ADDITION Lavender and calendula are herbs well known for their anti-inflammatory properties. To infuse these powerful herbs into your blend, steep 2 tablespoons each of lavender buds and calendula flowers in the coconut oil over low heat for 2 hours. Strain before using.

CALENDULA CHAMOMILE COMPRESS

MAKES 1 TREATMENT ❧ TOPICAL

2 tablespoons aloe vera gel

5 drops lavender essential oil

3 drops frankincense essential oil

2 drops neroli essential oil

4 cups boiling water

1. In a small bowl, stir together the aloe vera gel, and the lavender, frankincense, and neroli essential oils.
2. Add the hot water to a medium bowl, and stir in the aloe mixture.
3. To use, dip a washcloth into the mixture and wring it out. Apply to the forehead and feet to help draw heat from the body.

SUBSTITUTION TIP Anti-inflammatory chamomile makes a great substitution for the hot water in this recipe. Steep ½ cup of the herb in boiling water for 15 to 20 minutes before using in this recipe.

Blood Pressure

High blood pressure during pregnancy and labor can cause serious complications, including pre-eclampsia (see page 66). High blood pressure needs to be attended to by a medical doctor or midwife accordingly, but essential oils can help to calm the mind and relieve stress alongside the medical treatments. Stress-relieving and relaxing essential oils that help to calm the mind and body, such as lavender, chamomile, rosalina, bergamot, sweet orange, clary sage, coriander, marjoram, ylang-ylang, frankincense, mandarin, petitgrain, tangerine, cedarwood, sandalwood, vetiver, vanilla, and blue tansy, are perfect for the job.

RELAXING DELIVERY DIFFUSER BLEND #1
MAKES ½ OUNCE ❧ AROMATIC

1 teaspoon lavender essential oil
1 teaspoon sweet orange essential oil
¾ teaspoon Roman chamomile essential oil
25 drops ylang-ylang essential oil

1. Add all the essential oils to an empty essential oil bottle (or any dark glass bottle with a dropper) and gently swirl the bottle to combine.
2. Add 10 drops to a diffuser and diffuse throughout the room in 30-minute increments (30 minutes on/30 minutes off) to avoid overexposure.

RELAXING DELIVERY DIFFUSER BLEND #2
MAKES ½ OUNCE ❧ AROMATIC ❧ PHOTOSENSITIZING

1 teaspoon grapefruit essential oil
¾ teaspoon coriander essential oil
¾ teaspoon lemon essential oil
½ teaspoon Roman chamomile essential oil

1. Add all the essential oils to an empty essential oil bottle (or any dark glass bottle with a dropper) and gently swirl the bottle to combine.
2. Add 10 drops to a diffuser and diffuse throughout the room in 30-minute increments (30 minutes on/30 minutes off) to avoid overexposure.

HELPFUL HINT Dilute the blend in coconut oil or your favorite unscented lotion, and rub all over your body. Since this blend contains photosensitizing grapefruit and lemon oils, don't forget to dilute before using topically, and use caution in the sun.

Contractions

Aromatherapy helps you concentrate and focus during contractions, calms your mind and body, and prepares you for the next stage in your labor. Clary sage is especially effective at strengthening contractions and making them more effective. It is a favorite among midwives to use during labor. Other essential oils that can help you through the contractions include lavender, rosalina, chamomile, petitgrain, fir needle, cypress, spearmint, sweet orange, lemon, coriander, cedarwood, frankincense, patchouli, lemon eucalyptus, juniper berry, bergamot, and grapefruit.

BREATHE BABY MASSAGE OIL
MAKES 4 OUNCES ⁂ TOPICAL ⁂ AROMATIC

½ cup unrefined coconut oil

25 drops clary sage essential oil

20 drops lavender essential oil

20 drops rosalina essential oil

1. In a small pan over low heat, melt the coconut oil.
2. Once melted, remove from heat, add the clary sage, lavender, and rosalina essential oils, and stir to combine.
3. Pour into a Mason jar, and put into the freezer for 20 minutes to harden. (Store any unused oil in a cool, dark location.)
4. To use, apply to your chest, neck, temples, and the bottoms of your feet in between contractions.

YOU CAN DO IT DIFFUSER BLEND
MAKES ½ OUNCE ⁂ AROMATIC

1 teaspoon lavender essential oil

¾ teaspoon Atlas cedarwood essential oil

¾ teaspoon sweet orange essential oil

½ teaspoon clary sage essential oil

1. Add all the essential oils to an empty essential oil bottle (or any dark glass bottle with a dropper) and gently swirl the bottle to combine.
2. Add 10 drops to a diffuser and diffuse throughout the room in 30-minute increments (30 minutes on/30 minutes off) to avoid overexposure.

C-Section Care

With my medical conditions, I had no choice in my birth. I went through my pregnancy knowing that I would not get the normal birthing experience, but prepared myself in the areas that I had control over. Recovering from a C-section is different than natural birth recovery, but oftentimes healing can be handled with herbs and essential oils. Antibacterial skin and scar-healing essential oils such as lavender, chamomile, geranium, palmarosa, lemon, sweet orange, tangerine, neroli, frankincense, cedarwood, helichrysum can help heal up the scar while also calming nerves and soothing emotions in the hospital room.

HEALING C-SECTION SALVE

MAKES 4 OUNCES ≫ TOPICAL

¼ cup unrefined coconut oil
2 tablespoons beeswax pastilles
2 tablespoons tamanu oil
1 teaspoon vitamin E oil

30 drops lavender essential oil
20 drops frankincense essential oil
15 drops neroli essential oil

1. In a small pan over low heat, melt the coconut oil and beeswax.

2. Once melted, remove from heat, and add the tamanu oil, vitamin E, and the lavender, frankincense, and neroli essential oils.

3. Pour into a Mason jar, and put into the freezer for 20 minutes to harden.

4. Apply twice daily to your incision area. Store any unused salve in a cool, dark location.

AWESOME ADDITION Calendula and marshmallow root are herbs well known for their skin- and scar-healing properties. They would make a great addition to this salve. Steep 1 tablespoon each in the coconut oil over low heat for a couple hours. Strain before using in this recipe.

ANTIBACTERIAL C-SECTION WASH

MAKES 4 OUNCES ⅀ TOPICAL

2 tablespoons witch hazel
1 tablespoon aloe vera gel
½ teaspoon vegetable glycerin
10 drops lavender essential oil

10 drops tea tree essential oil
5 drops lemon essential oil
Filtered water, to fill

1. Combine the witch hazel, aloe vera gel, vegetable glycerin, and the lavender, tea tree, and lemon essential oils in a 4-ounce spray bottle. Gently swirl the bottle to combine.

2. Fill with the filtered water.

3. To use, spray onto the incision area and gently pat dry with a clean cloth or towel. Follow with Healing C-Section Salve (page 91). Store any unused spray in a cool, dark location.

SUBSTITUTION TIP For skin- and scar-healing benefits, substitute calendula or chamomile hydrosol for the water in this recipe. Both chamomile and calendula are well known to soothe inflammation, boost tissue regeneration, and heal wounds.

AFTER-THE-C DIFFUSER BLEND

MAKES ½ OUNCE ⅀ TOPICAL

1 teaspoon grapefruit essential oil
¾ teaspoon lavender essential oil

¾ teaspoon sweet orange essential oil
½ teaspoon clary sage essential oil

1. Add all the essential oils to an empty essential oil bottle (or any dark glass bottle with a dropper) and gently swirl the bottle to combine.

2. Add 10 drops to a diffuser and diffuse throughout the room in 30-minute increments (30 minutes on/30 minutes off) to avoid overexposure.

Episiotomy Care

An *episiotomy* is a surgical cut made to enlarge the vaginal opening before birth. It is usually performed to prevent tearing during the delivery of the baby. The area around the incision will be uncomfortable and sensitive for a few days. Cold packs, sitz baths, and a cleansing spray can help it heal up naturally. If you received stitches, only take one sitz bath a day until the stitches are removed. Antibacterial and anti-inflammatory essential oils including lavender, tea tree, chamomile, marjoram, geranium, palmarosa, lemon, sweet orange, tangerine, neroli, frankincense, cypress, fir needle, cedarwood, helichrysum, patchouli, and sandalwood all help to soothe inflamed skin and heal wounds.

HEALING EPISIOTOMY SALVE
MAKES 4 OUNCES ❧ TOPICAL

¼ cup unrefined coconut oil
2 tablespoons extra-virgin olive oil
2 tablespoons beeswax pastilles

30 drops lavender essential oil
20 drops German chamomile essential oil
20 drops marjoram essential oil

1. In a small pan over low heat, heat the coconut oil, olive oil, and beeswax.
2. Once melted, remove from the heat, and add the lavender, German chamomile, and marjoram essential oils.
3. Pour into a Mason jar, and put into the freezer for 20 minutes to harden.
4. Apply the salve to the episiotomy site after cleansing or when pain relief is needed. Store any unused salve in a cool, dark location.

ANTIBACTERIAL EPISIOTOMY WASH
MAKES 4 OUNCES ❧ TOPICAL

2 tablespoons witch hazel
1 tablespoon aloe vera gel
1 teaspoon vegetable glycerin

20 drops lavender essential oil
5 drops geranium essential oil
Filtered water, to fill

1. In a 4-ounce spray bottle, combine the witch hazel, aloe vera gel, and vegetable glycerin with the lavender and geranium essential oils. Gently swirl the bottle to mix.
2. Top off with the filtered water and swirl again to thoroughly combine.
3. To use, spray onto the episiotomy area and gently pat dry with a clean cloth or towel. Follow with Healing Episiotomy Salve (above). Store any unused wash in a cool, dark location.

SUBSTITUTION TIP For extra skin- and scar-healing benefits, substitute calendula or chamomile hydrosol for the water in this recipe. Both are well known for their abilities to soothe inflammation, boost tissue regeneration, and heal wounds.

HEALING AFTER-EPI SITZ BATH

MAKES 1 TREATMENT ⤳ TOPICAL

¼ cup aloe vera gel

6 drops lavender essential oil

3 drops cypress essential oil

1 cup Epsom salt

1. In a small bowl, stir together the aloe vera and the lavender and cypress essential oils.

2. Place the Epsom salt in a medium bowl and stir in the aloe vera mixture.

3. Pour the mixture under the running bath water, filling the tub quarter to half full.

4. Sit in the bath and soak the bottom half of your body for at least 20 minutes.

AWESOME ADDITION Soothing antibacterial herbs such as lavender and calendula make great additions to this sitz bath. Add ½ cup of each herb to a cloth tea bag or an old, clean sock, and tie closed before tossing into the bathtub.

Fatigue During Labor

Giving birth is hard work, and it's quite natural to run out of energy during labor. Aromatherapy has many benefits to the laboring mother. Uplifting essential oils such as lemon, grapefruit, coriander, fir needle, palmarosa, ginger, cedarwood, petitgrain, tangerine, spruce, spearmint, juniper berry, geranium, pine, sweet orange, black pepper, and bergamot can cleanse the air, brighten the mood, and boost energy when you need it the most to help you power through the tough parts with a little more oomph.

ENERGY BUILDER DIFFUSER BLEND

MAKES ½ OUNCE ⤳ AROMATIC ⤳ PHOTOSENSITIZING

1 teaspoon spearmint essential oil

¾ teaspoon bergamot essential oil

¾ teaspoon sweet orange essential oil

½ teaspoon lemon essential oil

1. Add all the essential oils to an empty essential oil bottle (or any dark glass bottle with a dropper), and gently swirl the bottle to combine.

2. Add 10 drops to a diffuser and diffuse throughout the room in 30-minute increments (30 minutes on/30 minutes off) at a time to avoid overexposure.

HELPFUL HINT Dilute this blend in coconut oil or your favorite unscented lotion and massage onto your chest, shoulders, hands, and feet. Bergamot and lemon essential oils are photosensitizing, so don't forget to dilute before using topically, and use caution in the sun.

HIGH ENERGY AROMATHERAPY INHALER
MAKES ⅓ OUNCE ❧ AROMATIC

15 drops tangerine essential oil
5 drops Atlas cedarwood essential oil

5 drops ginger essential oil
5 drops palmarosa essential oil

1. Combine all the essential oils in a small glass bowl.
2. Using tweezers, add the wick (the cotton pad) of an aromatherapy personal inhaler to the bowl and roll it around until it's soaked up all of the essential oils mixture.
3. Use the tweezers to transfer the wick to the inhaler tube. Close the tube and label the inhaler.
4. Take a whiff of the inhaler whenever you need a boost of energy.

ENERGIZING AROMATHERAPY ROOM SPRAY
MAKES 6 OUNCES ❧ AROMATIC

5 ounces filtered water
2 tablespoons 80-proof vodka
30 drops spruce essential oil

25 drops tangerine essential oil
15 drops lemon essential oil
10 drops petitgrain essential oil

1. Add all the ingredients to a spray bottle and shake to combine.
2. Spray around the room and on pillows and furniture to enjoy the scent throughout the room.

SUBSTITUTION TIP If you don't have vodka on hand, witch hazel makes a great substitute in a room spray. Be sure to shake the bottle well before spraying. Witch hazel contains only a small percentage of alcohol and the essential oils will not mix into the water like they would with vodka.

Germ Killing

When newborns arrive in this world, they have no protection against infections and viruses. Breastfeeding for at least one week helps infants build their immune system, but essential oils can help with neutralizing germs in the air and from guests. Antiseptic, antibacterial, and antiviral essential oils include lavender, tea tree, lemon, sweet orange, grapefruit, tangerine, mandarin, marjoram, chamomile, palmarosa, fir needle, cypress, frankincense, geranium, coriander, bergamot, cedarwood, helichrysum, rosalina, neroli, petitgrain, and sandalwood.

ANTIBACTERIAL HAND GEL
MAKES 1 OUNCE

2 tablespoons aloe vera gel

8 drops lavender essential oil

5 drops lemon essential oil

5 drops tea tree essential oil

1. Combine all the ingredients in a bottle and shake well to combine.

2. To use, squeeze a small amount of gel onto hands and rub in.

SAFETY TIP For a kid-safe version (2+ years), use half the drops of essential oil called for in this recipe. Label the junior version for any children who might come to visit the newest family member.

ANTIBACTERIAL FOAMING HAND SOAP
MAKES 8 OUNCES ≫ TOPICAL

1 tablespoon liquid castile soap

1 tablespoon vegetable glycerin

5 drops lavender essential oil

5 drops rosalina essential oil

¾ cup plus 2 tablespoons
   filtered water

1. In a foaming hand soap dispenser, combine liquid castile soap, vegetable glycerin, and the lavender and rosalina essential oils. Gently swirl the bottle to combine.

2. Fill with the filtered water, and seal. Shake well to combine the mixture.

SUBSTITUTION TIP For extra-gentle antibacterial benefits, substitute lavender hydrosol for the water in this remedy. Lavender is well known for its abilities to soothe inflammation, cleanse a wound, and heal dry skin.

GERM-KILLING DIFFUSER BLEND
MAKES ½ OUNCE ≫ AROMATIC

1 teaspoon sweet orange essential oil

¾ teaspoon lavender essential oil

¾ teaspoon rosalina essential oil

½ teaspoon palmarosa essential oil

1. Add all the essential oils to an empty essential oil bottle (or any dark glass bottle with a dropper), and gently swirl the bottle to combine.

2. Add 10 drops to a diffuser and diffuse throughout the room in 30-minute increments (30 minutes on/30 minutes off) to avoid overexposure.

Hair Loss

After giving birth, hormone levels fluctuate while you produce food for your baby and your torso shrinks back to pre-pregnancy size. You may experience postpartum hair thinning or hair falling out because of this. But don't worry, because hair loss typically stops within 6 to 9 months of birth. Essential oils such as lavender, cedarwood, clary sage, chamomile, lemon, spearmint, patchouli, tea tree, vetiver, ylang-ylang, cypress, fir needle, juniper berry, pine, sweet orange, sandalwood, coriander, geranium, frankincense, and black pepper can help support hair health.

HERBAL GODDESS HAIR GROWTH SERUM
MAKES 4 OUNCES ≫ TOPICAL

½ cup castor oil

1 tablespoon rosemary

1 tablespoon horsetail

15 drops lavender essential oil

10 drops clary sage essential oil

10 drops geranium essential oil

1. Combine the castor oil and herbs in a small pan, cover, and bring to a simmer over low heat. Remove from heat and allow to steep covered, for 2 hours.

2. Strain the oil into a Mason jar, and add the lavender, clary sage, and geranium essential oils.

3. To use, massage a dime-size amount onto your scalp and roots.

4. Follow with a boar-bristle brush and brush hair from roots to ends. Store any unused serum in a cool, dark location.

HAIR GROWTH DETANGLING SPRAY
MAKES 8 OUNCES ➤ TOPICAL

¾ cup filtered water

2 tablespoons aloe vera gel

2 tablespoons castor oil

10 drops Atlas cedarwood essential oil

10 drops lavender essential oil

1. Combine all the ingredients in an 8-ounce glass spray bottle and shake well.

2. Spray onto hair before combing through.

AWESOME ADDITIONS You can make this hair growth detangling spray even more amazing by first steeping lavender and rosemary in the castor oil before using in the recipe. You can also substitute rosemary or lavender hydrosol for the filtered water.

SIMPLE HAIR GROWTH SCALP MASSAGE OIL
MAKES 2 OUNCES ➤ TOPICAL

¼ cup castor oil

15 drops lavender essential oil

10 drops cypress essential oil

1. Combine all the ingredients in a bottle, and gently swirl to combine.

2. Massage a dime-size amount of the oil into the scalp and pull through your hair to the ends.

Milk Production

While some breastfeeding mamas have no trouble producing milk, others, like myself, have to work to produce enough milk for our babies. Good nutrition and feeding baby often are keys to producing milk, but there are herbs and essential oils that can help when that is not enough. Drinking teas made with herbs that are *galactagogues* (substances that encourage milk production), such as alfalfa, blessed thistle, fennel, fenugreek, and dandelion, can help increase your milk supply. Applying essential oils of clary sage and geranium topically can also help stimulate milk production. Note that although many books and websites suggest fennel essential oil increases milk supply, new studies now show that fennel essential oil is estrogenic, making it inadvisable to use in any way while pregnant, nursing, around children younger than 6 years old, or even around women with endometriosis. Fennel tea is far less concentrated and is safe to use instead.

MORE MILK MASSAGE OIL
MAKES 2 OUNCES ⇒ TOPICAL

¼ cup extra-virgin olive oil
10 drops clary sage essential oil

10 drops geranium essential oil

1. Add all the ingredients to a dark glass bottle, and gently swirl to combine.
2. To use, massage oil into breasts in a circular motion, avoiding the nipple area.

AWESOME ADDITION Fennel seeds are well known for their galactagogic properties and would make a great addition to this oil. Steep 2 tablespoons fennel seeds in the olive oil over low heat for 2 hours. Strain before using in this recipe.

MILK MAMA HERBAL LINIMENT
MAKES 1 TREATMENT ⇒ TOPICAL

1 cup 80-proof vodka
¼ cup fennel seeds, crushed
¼ cup fenugreek seeds, crushed

10 drops geranium essential oil
10 drops clary sage essential oil

1. Combine all the ingredients in a Mason jar. Cover and steep on the kitchen counter for 2 weeks. Shake the jar twice a day to mix the contents.
2. Strain the mixture into a spray bottle.
3. To use, spray onto your breasts and allow it to sink in.

SUBSTITUTION TIP Witch hazel can be substituted for the vodka in this recipe. Be sure to shake the bottle well before spraying. Witch hazel contains only a small percentage of alcohol and the essential oils will not mix into the witch hazel like they would with vodka.

Nausea

Nausea and vomiting are common during labor, especially during the transition phase. It is important to hydrate as often as possible, and herbal teas count as a great source of hydration and valuable nutrients. Lemons are a natural source of electrolytes, vitamin C, and antioxidants. Fresh lemon and ginger tea can help keep you hydrated and soothe your nauseated stomach at the same time. Digestive essential oils such as ginger, spearmint, chamomile, lemon, sweet orange, grapefruit, bergamot, mandarin, tangerine, and dill weed can all be used to help alleviate nausea and vomiting during labor as well.

TUMMY TAMER AROMATHERAPY ROLL-ON
MAKES ⅓ OUNCE ☞ TOPICAL

3 drops ginger essential oil
2 drops spearmint essential oil

1 drop Roman chamomile essential oil
Fractionated coconut oil

1. Add the ginger, spearmint, and Roman chamomile essential oils to a ⅓-ounce glass roll-on bottle, then fill the bottle with the fractionated coconut oil. Seal the bottle, and gently swirl to combine. Don't forget to label your creation.
2. To use, roll onto the back of your neck, chest, and wrists whenever you are feeling anxious or stressed.

SOOTHING ANTI-NAUSEA DIFFUSER BLEND
MAKES ½ OUNCE ☞ AROMATIC

1 teaspoon sweet orange essential oil
¾ teaspoon ginger essential oil

¾ teaspoon Roman chamomile essential oil
½ teaspoon petitgrain essential oil

1. Add all the essential oils to an empty essential oil bottle (or any dark glass bottle with a dropper), and gently swirl the bottle to combine.
2. Add 10 drops to a diffuser and diffuse throughout the room in 30-minute increments (30 minutes on/30 minutes off) at a time to avoid overexposure.

HELPFUL TIP Dilute the blend in coconut oil or your favorite unscented lotion, and apply to your stomach, chest, and neck.

NIX THE NAUSEA AROMATHERAPY INHALER
MAKES 1 TREATMENT ➢ AROMATIC

10 drops lemon essential oil

10 drops sweet orange essential oil

5 drops petitgrain essential oil

5 drops Roman chamomile essential oil

1. Combine all the essential oils in a small glass bowl.
2. Using tweezers, add the wick (the cotton pad) of an aromatherapy personal inhaler to the bowl. Roll it around until it's soaked up all of the essential oils mixture.
3. Use the tweezers to transfer the wick to the inhaler tube. Close the tube and label the inhaler.
4. Take a whiff of the inhaler whenever you are feeling nauseated.

Nipples, Dry/Cracked

How well your nipples fare while nursing can depend on whether your baby is latching on correctly. If your baby is taking too much breast into their mouth, your nipples will pay the price. A trained lactation specialist can help you with latching and any other nursing needs. Gentle essential oils such as lavender, chamomile, geranium, neroli, blue tansy, helichrysum, sweet orange, and rose will help to soothe inflammation and heal any open wounds.

MAMA'S BOOBIE BALM
MAKES 4 OUNCES ➢ TOPICAL

¼ cup unrefined coconut oil

2 tablespoons beeswax pastilles

2 tablespoons unrefined shea butter

30 drops German chamomile essential oil

1. In a small pan over low heat, melt the coconut oil, beeswax, and shea butter.
2. Once melted, remove from heat, and add the German chamomile essential oil. ➔

3. Pour into a Mason jar, and put into the freezer for 20 minutes to harden.

4. After breastfeeding, gently pat your nipples dry and apply the balm to prevent future nipple damage. You can also apply to both breasts whenever relief is needed. Store any unused balm in a cool, dark location.

AWESOME ADDITION Calendula flowers are well known for their anti-inflammatory and antibacterial properties. I never make a skin-healing salve without them. Steep 2 tablespoons of calendula in the coconut oil over low heat for 2 hours. Strain before using in this recipe.

HERBAL-INFUSED HEALING NIPPLE OIL
MAKES 4 OUNCES ❧ TOPICAL

½ cup extra-virgin olive oil

2 tablespoons calendula flowers

2 tablespoons lavender buds

20 drops lavender essential oil

10 drops geranium essential oil

1. Combine all the ingredients in a glass bowl. Pour into a Mason jar.

2. After breastfeeding, gently pat nipples dry and apply the oil to prevent future nipple damage. You can also apply to both breasts whenever relief is needed.

3. Store any unused oil in a cool, dark location.

Postpartum Depression

Because of the massive fluctuation in hormones during and after pregnancy, many women experience some form of postpartum depression, though some may not know it. It is important to consult your medical practitioner if you think you may be experiencing depression. There are both natural and pharmaceutical treatments that can help. Essential oils that are helpful at relieving stress and anxiety, and boosting the mood, alongside any medical treatments, include lavender, chamomile, clary sage, lemon, sweet orange, grapefruit, petitgrain, geranium, coriander, bergamot, vanilla, sandalwood, ylang-ylang, cedarwood, and neroli.

CHEER UP SUNSHINE DIFFUSER BLEND

MAKES ½ OUNCE ❧ AROMATIC ❧ PHOTOSENSITIZING

1 teaspoon sweet orange essential oil
¾ teaspoon bergamot essential oil

¾ teaspoon lavender essential oil
½ teaspoon coriander essential oil

1. Add all the essential oils to an empty essential oil bottle (or any dark glass bottle with a dropper), and gently swirl the bottle to combine.

2. Add 10 drops to a diffuser and diffuse throughout the room in 30-minute increments (30 minutes on/30 minutes off) at a time to avoid overexposure.

HELPFUL HINT Dilute the blend in coconut oil or in your favorite unscented lotion and massage all over your body. This blend contains photosensitizing bergamot oil, so don't forget to dilute before using topically, and use caution in the sun.

BEAT THE BABY BLUES BODY SPRAY

MAKES 4 OUNCES ❧ TOPICAL

2 tablespoons witch hazel
1½ teaspoons aloe vera gel
½ teaspoon vegetable glycerin
25 drops clary sage essential oil

20 drops Roman chamomile essential oil
15 drops sandalwood essential oil
Filtered water, to fill

1. In a 4-ounce spray bottle, combine the witch hazel, aloe vera gel, and vegetable glycerin with the clary sage, Roman chamomile, and sandalwood essential oils. Gently swirl the bottle to mix.

2. Fill the bottle with the filtered water.

3. Shake well before use. Spray onto your hair and body. Store any unused spray in a cool, dark location.

HELPFUL HINT This blend can be used as a room and pillow spray, too. Spray around the room and on pillows and furniture to enjoy the scent throughout the room.

BLUES BUSTER AROMATHERAPY ROLL-ON

MAKES ⅓ OUNCE ≫ TOPICAL ≫ PHOTOSENSITIZING

3 drops bergamot essential oil

2 drops Roman chamomile essential oil

1 drop frankincense essential oil

Fractionated coconut oil

1. Add the bergamot, Roman chamomile, and frankincense essential oils to a ⅓-ounce glass roll-on bottle.
2. Fill the bottle with the fractionated coconut oil. Place the roller ball and cap on and gently swirl to combine. Label your creation.
3. To use, roll onto the back of your neck, chest, and wrists whenever you are feeling depressed, anxious, or stressed.

Postpartum Vaginal Care

By this point, your vagina has been through a lot, but with a little care you can return to your pre-pregnancy self in no time. Healing compresses, antibacterial washes, and sitz baths can all help to reduce inflammation and soothe any residual pain. Antibacterial and anti-inflammatory essential oils including lavender, tea tree, chamomile, marjoram, geranium, palmarosa, lemon, sweet orange, tangerine, neroli, frankincense, cypress, fir needle, cedarwood, helichrysum, patchouli, and sandalwood all help to soothe inflammation and heal wounds.

HEALING VAGINAL COMPRESS

MAKES 1 TREATMENT ≫ TOPICAL

5 drops lavender essential oil

3 drops geranium essential oil

2 tablespoons aloe vera gel

1 cup witch hazel

4 cups boiling water

1. In a small bowl, stir together the lavender and geranium essential oils with the aloe vera gel.
2. Add the witch hazel to a medium bowl and stir in the aloe mixture.
3. Fill the bowl with hot water, leaving room to dip a washcloth in it without overflow.
4. To use, dip a washcloth into the mixture and wring it out. Apply to the vagina, perineum, and anus for relief.

SUBSTITUTION TIP Anti-inflammatory chamomile makes a great substitute for the water in this recipe. Steep ½ cup of the herb in boiling water for 15 to 20 minutes before using.

POSTPARTUM VAGINAL WIPES
MAKES 24 WIPES ⤳ TOPICAL

1 tablespoon unrefined coconut oil

5 drops helichrysum essential oil

5 drops lavender essential oil

½ cup witch hazel

1. In a small pan over low heat, melt the coconut oil. Add the helichrysum and lavender essential oils and stir to combine.
2. Pour the witch hazel into a medium bowl. Whisk the coconut oil mixture into the witch hazel.
3. Cut 12 paper towels in half and stack them in a glass container that has a lid. Pour over the stack of paper towels. The paper towels should soak up all the liquid.
4. Cover the wipes with the lid and store in the refrigerator when not using for up to 1 month.

POSTPARTUM SITZ BATH
MAKES 1 TREATMENT ⤳ TOPICAL

5 drops lavender essential oil

5 drops German chamomile essential oil

¼ cup aloe vera gel

1 cup Epsom salt

1. In a small bowl, stir together the lavender and German chamomile essential oils with the aloe vera gel.
2. Place the Epsom salt in a medium bowl and stir in the aloe vera mixture.
3. Pour the mixture under running bath water, filling the tub quarter to half full.
4. Sit in the bath and soak the bottom half of your body for at least 20 minutes.

AWESOME ADDITION Soothing herbs such as lavender and oats make great additions to this sitz bath. Add ½ cup of each to a cloth tea bag or an old, clean sock, and tie closed before tossing into the bathtub.

Sore Breasts

One of the number one complaints of breastfeeding mamas is sore breasts. Warm compresses and massage oils can help soothe the pain and give you relief. Anti-inflammatory and pain-relieving essential oils including lavender, chamomile, rosalina, petitgrain, ginger, marjoram, helichrysum, sandalwood, frankincense, ylang-ylang, patchouli, blue tansy, and geranium can also help to relieve some of the pain.

SORE BREAST MASSAGE OIL
MAKES 4 OUNCES ⨾ TOPICAL

½ cup unrefined coconut oil

30 drops lavender essential oil

22 drops rosalina essential oil

20 drops Roman chamomile essential oil

1. In a small pan over low heat, melt the coconut oil.
2. Once melted, remove from heat, add the lavender, rosalina, and Roman chamomile essential oils, and stir to combine.
3. Pour into a Mason jar, and put into the freezer for 20 minutes to harden.
4. Apply a small amount to the area that aches and massage in. Store any unused oil in a cool, dark location.

AWESOME ADDITION Arnica flowers and St. John's wort are herbs well known for their anti-inflammatory properties and make a great addition to any pain relief oil or salve. Steep 2 tablespoons of each herb in the coconut oil over low heat for 2 hours. Strain before using in this recipe.

ANTI-INFLAMMATORY HERBAL BREAST COMPRESS

MAKES 1 TREATMENT ≫ TOPICAL

2 tablespoons aloe vera gel

5 drops lavender essential oil

5 drops Roman chamomile essential oil

Hot water

1. Combine the aloe vera gel and essential oils together in a medium glass bowl.
2. Fill the bowl with hot water, leaving room to dip a washcloth in it without overflow.
3. To use, dip a washcloth into the mixture, and wring out the excess. Apply to the breasts as often as needed for relief.

SUBSTITUTION TIP Lavender tea is well known for its gentle anti-inflammatory properties and makes a great substitution for the hot water in this recipe. Steep ½ cup of the herb in boiling water for 15 to 20 minutes before using in this recipe.

Speed Up Labor

While I generally do not promote inducing labor, I do believe when labor stalls, a little push from aromatherapy can get labor going again. Clary sage essential oil is well known for its ability to make contractions more effective. The easiest way to use it during labor is to put a couple drops on a washcloth and inhale it in between contractions, but I prefer to diffuse it throughout the room or use it in a personal aromatherapy inhaler. Other essential oils that get things moving along during labor are cypress, fir needle, juniper berry, lavender, coriander, frankincense, rosalina, geranium, jasmine, rose, and ylang-ylang.

GET THINGS GOING DIFFUSER BLEND
MAKES ½ OUNCE ❧ AROMATIC

1¼ teaspoons clary sage essential oil
1 teaspoon lemon essential oil

¾ teaspoon geranium
    essential oil

1. Add all the essential oils to an empty essential oil bottle (or any dark glass bottle with a dropper) and gently swirl the bottle to combine.
2. Add 10 drops to a diffuser and diffuse throughout the room in 30-minute increments (30 minutes on/30 minutes off) at a time to avoid overexposure.

STALLED LABOR AROMATHERAPY INHALER
MAKES 1 TREATMENT ❧ AROMATIC

10 drops clary sage essential oil
10 drops jasmine absolute

10 drops lavender
    essential oil

1. Combine all the essential oils in a small glass bowl.
2. Using tweezers, add the wick (the cotton pad) of an aromatherapy personal inhaler to the bowl and roll it around until it's soaked up all of the essential oils mixture.
3. Use the tweezers to transfer the wick to the inhaler tube. Close the tube and label the inhaler.
4. Take a whiff of the inhaler whenever needed during your labor.

Transition

Though it is truly the calm before the storm and the shortest stage of labor, many would call transition labor the hardest part of birthing. Many women experience feelings of anxiety and fear as well as nausea, chills, stronger contractions, the urge to push, and possibly even the rupturing of membranes. Aromatherapy can freshen the delivery room, calm anxieties, and keep labor on track. Use bright and calming essential oils such as lavender, chamomile, clary sage, coriander, lemon, sweet orange, bergamot, tangerine, mandarin, vanilla, and frankincense.

TRANSITION AROMATHERAPY ROOM SPRAY

MAKES 6 OUNCES ⇒ AROMATIC

5 ounces filtered water
2 tablespoons 80-proof vodka
20 drops grapefruit essential oil

15 drops clary sage essential oil
15 drops tangerine essential oil
10 drops lavender essential oil

1. Add all the ingredients to a spray bottle and shake to combine.
2. Spray around the room and on pillows and furniture to enjoy the scent throughout the room.

SUBSTITUTION TIP If you don't have vodka on hand, witch hazel makes a great substitute in a room spray. Be sure to shake the bottle well before spraying. Witch hazel contains only a small percentage of alcohol and the essential oils will not mix into the water like they would with vodka.

TRANSITION AROMATHERAPY ROLL-ON

MAKES ⅓ OUNCE ⇒ TOPICAL ⇒ AROMATIC

2 drops lavender essential oil
2 drops Roman chamomile essential oil
2 drops tangerine essential oil

1 drop vanilla CO_2 (12%)
Fractionated coconut oil

1. Add the essential oils to a ⅓-ounce glass roll-on bottle then add fractionated coconut oil to fill. Place the roller ball and cap on and gently swirl to combine. Don't forget to label your creation.
2. To use, roll onto the back of your neck, chest, and wrists as needed.

TRANSITION DIFFUSER BLEND

MAKES ½ OUNCE ⇒ AROMATIC

1 teaspoon lavender essential oil
1 teaspoon Roman chamomile
  essential oil

¾ teaspoon tangerine essential oil
25 drops vanilla CO_2 (12%)

1. Add all the essential oils to an empty essential oil bottle (or any dark glass bottle with a dropper), and gently swirl the bottle to combine.
2. Add 10 drops to a diffuser and diffuse throughout the room in 30-minute increments (30 minutes on/30 minutes off) to avoid overexposure.

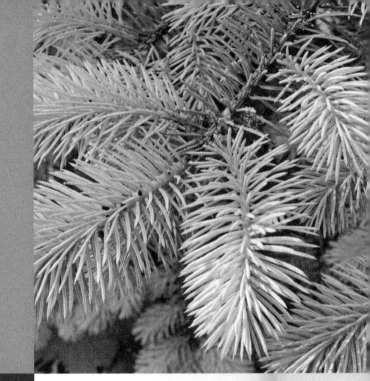

CHAPTER
FIVE

Blends for Infants
& Young Children

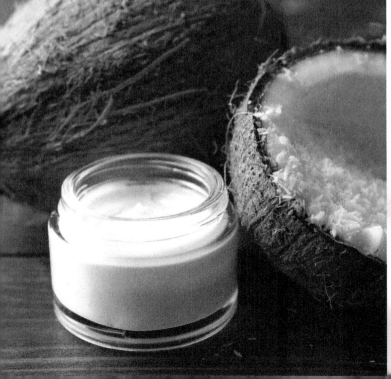

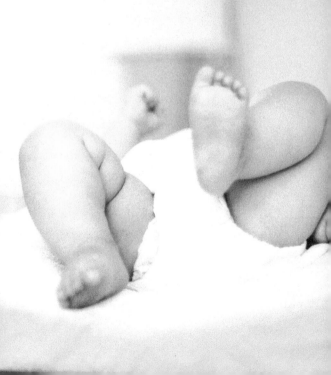

Allergies (Hay Fever)

Allergies can strike any time of year, depending on what your child is allergic to. Many over-the-counter allergy medications have unwanted side effects, such as drowsiness and irritability. Aromatherapy is a great tool against hay fever, helping to cleanse and purify the air we breathe, soothing irritated sinus passage membranes, and opening up airways for better breathing. Essential oils that soothe allergies and sinus issues include lavender, blue tansy, chamomile, lemon, frankincense, sweet orange, grapefruit, juniper berry, spearmint, spruce, fir needle, cypress, pine, rosalina, citronella, and lemon eucalyptus.

ALLERGY ANNIHILATOR DIFFUSER BLEND #1

MAKES ½ OUNCE ⫶ AROMATIC

1 teaspoon fir needle essential oil

1 teaspoon rosalina essential oil

¾ teaspoon blue tansy essential oil

¾ teaspoon German chamomile essential oil

TO MAKE THE BLEND

Add all the essential oils to an empty essential oil bottle (or any dark glass bottle with a dropper) and gently swirl the bottle to combine.

TO DIFFUSE THE BLEND

Add the recommended drops to a diffuser and diffuse throughout the room in 30-minute increments (30 minutes on/30 minutes off).

0–6 mo.	6–24 mo.	2–6 yr.	6+ yr.
2 drops	4 drops	6 drops	8 drops

ALLERGY ANNIHILATOR DIFFUSER BLEND #2

MAKES ½ OUNCE >< AROMATIC

1 teaspoon rosalina essential oil

¾ teaspoon fir needle essential oil

¾ teaspoon lavender essential oil

½ teaspoon lemon essential oil

TO MAKE THE BLEND

Add all the essential oils to an empty essential oil bottle (or any dark glass bottle with a dropper), and gently swirl the bottle to combine.

TO DIFFUSE THE BLEND

Add the recommended drops to a diffuser and diffuse throughout the room in 30-minute increments (30 minutes on/30 minutes off).

0–6 mo.	6–24 mo.	2–6 yr.	6+ yr.
2 drops	4 drops	6 drops	8 drops

HAY FEVER AROMATHERAPY INHALER

MAKES 1 TREATMENT >< AROMATIC

	3–6 mo.	6–24 mo.	2–6 yr.	6+ yr.
Blue tansy essential oil	no drops	3 drops	6 drops	6 drops
Lemon essential oil	6 drops	3 drops	6 drops	6 drops
Rosalina essential oil	4 drops	4 drops	8 drops	8 drops

1. Combine all the essential oils in a small glass bowl.
2. Using tweezers, add the wick (the cotton pad) of an aromatherapy personal inhaler to the bowl and roll it around until it's soaked up all of the essential oils mixture.
3. Use the tweezers to transfer the wick to the inhaler tube. Close the tube and label the inhaler.
4. Use the inhaler whenever seasonal allergies start.

Anxiety

Children can have anxiety for many reasons, so it's important to teach them techniques to calm their anxious minds early on in their lives. Teaching children yoga and meditation are great tools. In addition, calming and stress-relieving essential oils such as lavender, chamomile, rosalina, petitgrain, neroli, cedarwood, ylang-ylang, lemon, sweet orange, bergamot, grapefruit, mandarin, rose, sandalwood, coriander, frankincense, and vanillas can help to reduce anxiety and work well alongside medical treatments.

ANTI-ANXIETY DIFFUSER BLEND

MAKES ½ OUNCE ⇒ AROMATIC

1 teaspoon lavender essential oil

¾ teaspoon grapefruit essential oil

¾ teaspoon sweet orange essential oil

½ teaspoon coriander essential oil

TO MAKE THE BLEND

Add all the essential oils to an empty essential oil bottle (or any dark glass bottle with a dropper), and gently swirl the bottle to combine.

TO DIFFUSE THE BLEND

Add the recommended drops to a diffuser and diffuse throughout the room in 30-minute increments (30 minutes on/30 minutes off).

0–6 mo.	6–24 mo.	2–6 yr.	6+ yr.
2 drops	4 drops	6 drops	8 drops

ANXIOUS CHILD MASSAGE OIL

MAKES ABOUT 2 OUNCES ⤳ TOPICAL

	3–6 mo.	6–24 mo.	2–6 yr.	6+ yr.
Carrier oil	¼ cup	¼ cup	¼ cup	¼ cup
Lavender essential oil	1 drop	6 drops	10 drops	15 drops
Roman chamomile essential oil	1 drop	4 drops	8 drops	15 drops

1. In a small pan over low heat, melt the carrier oil.
2. Once melted, remove from heat, and add the essential oils.
3. Combine the carrier oil and essential oils in a bottle or jar, and store in a cool, dark location when not in use.
4. Massage the oil onto your child's chest, back, legs, and the bottoms of their feet.

PEACEFUL BABY AROMATHERAPY ROOM SPRAY

MAKES 4 OUNCES ⤳ AROMATIC

	3–6 mo.	6–24 mo.	2–6 yr.	6+ yr.
Filtered water	3 oz.	3 oz.	3 oz.	3 oz.
80-proof vodka	2 tbsp.	2 tbsp.	2 tbsp.	2 tbsp.
Tangerine essential oil	2 drops	5 drops	10 drops	15 drops
Bergamot essential oil	no drops	5 drops	10 drops	15 drops
Lavender essential oil	2 drops	10 drops	15 drops	20 drops

1. Add all the ingredients to a spray bottle and shake to combine.
2. Spray around the room and on pillows and furniture to enjoy the scent throughout the room.

SUBSTITUTION TIP If you don't have vodka on hand, witch hazel makes a great substitute in a room spray. Be sure to shake the bottle well before spraying. Witch hazel contains only a small percentage of alcohol and the essential oils will not mix into the water like they would with vodka.

Asthma

According to the Asthma and Allergy Foundation of America, about 24 million Americans suffer from the respiratory condition, with children being the main sufferers. The condition strikes when the breathing pathways are irritated and become clogged with mucus, then constrict, making it difficult to breathe. Asthma can be life-threatening for some children, so be sure to consult your medical practitioner, but essential oils can safely accompany medication. Essential oils that help soothe irritation, reduce inflammation, open up airways, and cleanse the air include lavender, blue tansy, chamomile, lemon, frankincense, sweet orange, grapefruit, juniper berry, spearmint, spruce, fir needle, cypress, pine, rosalina, citronella, and lemon eucalyptus.

BREATHE BETTER DIFFUSER BLEND
MAKES ½ OUNCE ⁓ AROMATIC

1 teaspoon marjoram essential oil
1 teaspoon rosalina essential oil

½ teaspoon blue tansy essential oil
½ teaspoon fir needle essential oil

TO MAKE THE BLEND
Add all the essential oils to an empty essential oil bottle (or any dark glass bottle with a dropper), and gently swirl the bottle to combine.

TO DIFFUSE THE BLEND

Add the recommended drops to a diffuser and diffuse throughout the room in 30-minute increments (30 minutes on/30 minutes off).

0–6 mo.	6–24 mo.	2–6 yr.	6+ yr.
2 drops	4 drops	6 drops	8 drops

SUBSTITUTION TIP Blue tansy essential oil contains the chemical constituent azulene, a natural antihistamine that works well with allergies and asthma. If you do not have blue tansy on hand, German chamomile also contains azulene and can substitute for blue tansy (at a 1:1 ratio).

CALM BREATH AROMATHERAPY ROLL-ON
MAKES ABOUT ⅓ OUNCE ⋗ TOPICAL ⋗ AROMATIC

	3–6 mo.	6–24 mo.	2–6 yr.	6+ yr.
Frankincense essential oil	no drops	1 drop	1 drop	1 drop
Lavender essential oil	no drops	1 drop	1 drop	2 drops
Rosalina essential oil	no drops	1 drop	2 drops	3 drops
Fractionated coconut oil	to fill	to fill	to fill	to fill

1. Add the frankincense, lavender, and rosalina essential oils to a ⅓-ounce glass roll-on bottle.
2. Add enough fractionated coconut oil to fill the bottle. Place the roller ball and cap on and gently swirl to combine. Don't forget to label your creation.
3. To use, roll onto the back of the neck, chest, and wrists whenever breathing is difficult.

BREATHE EASY BEDTIME BATH

MAKES 1 TREATMENT ❧ TOPICAL ❧ AROMATIC

	3–6 mo.	6–24 mo.	2–6 yr.	6+ yr.
Fir needle essential oil	no drops	no drops	2 drops	2 drops
Lavender essential oil	2 drops	2 drops	2 drops	2 drops
Rosalina essential oil	no drops	2 drops	2 drops	2 drops
Unscented castile soap or baby shampoo	2 tbsp.	2 tbsp.	2 tbsp.	2 tbsp.
Epsom salt	1 cup	1 cup	1 cup	1 cup

1. In a small bowl, stir together the fir needle, lavender, and rosalina essential oils with the liquid soap

2. Place the Epsom salt in a medium bowl and stir in the soap mixture.

3. Pour the mixture under the running bath water as you fill the tub.

SUBSTITUTION TIP Instead of unscented soap, you can use your favorite carrier oil in this recipe, but be cautious when exiting because the oil will make the tub very slippery.

Athlete's Foot

Athlete's foot is a fungal infection that got its name from the many athletes who have picked it up from walking around barefoot in locker rooms and communal showers. Public pools, showers, gyms, and even yoga mats can be culprits. Soothing antifungal essential oils including lavender, tea tree, coriander, sweet orange, lemon, mandarin, grapefruit, tangerine, geranium, chamomile, pine, cedarwood, and frankincense can all combat fungi on the feet.

ANTIFUNGAL FOOT POWDER
MAKES ABOUT 1 CUP ❧ TOPICAL

	3–6 mo.	6–24 mo.	2–6 yr.	6+ yr.
White kaolin clay	½ cup	½ cup	½ cup	½ cup
Arrowroot powder or cornstarch	½ cup	½ cup	½ cup	½ cup
Geranium essential oil	no drops	no drops	5 drops	10 drops
Lavender essential oil	no drops	no drops	5 drops	10 drops
Tea tree essential oil	no drops	no drops	5 drops	10 drops

1. In a medium glass bowl, combine the clay, arrowroot powder, and essential oils.
2. Wash the affected area and dry thoroughly. Sprinkle a thin layer of the foot powder over the affected area twice daily (morning and night). Pay special attention to spaces between the toes and wear well-fitting, ventilated shoes. Change socks at least once daily.
3. Store foot powder in a Mason jar when not using.

FUNGUS AMUNGUS JR. SALVE

MAKES 4 OUNCES ❧ TOPICAL

	3–6 mo.	6–24 mo.	2–6 yr.	6+ yr.
Unrefined coconut oil	¼ cup	¼ cup	¼ cup	¼ cup
Beeswax pastilles	2 tbsp.	2 tbsp.	2 tbsp.	2 tbsp.
Unrefined shea butter	2 tbsp.	2 tbsp.	2 tbsp.	2 tbsp.
Lavender essential oil	2 drops	8 drops	15 drops	30 drops
Tea tree essential oil	2 drops	7 drops	10 drops	30 drops
Virginia cedarwood essential oil	no drops	5 drops	8 drops	10 drops

1. In a small pan over low heat, melt the coconut oil, beeswax, and shea butter.
2. Once melted, remove from heat, and add the lavender, tea tree, and Virginia cedarwood essential oils.
3. Pour into a Mason jar, and put into the freezer for 20 minutes to harden.
4. Apply the salve to any fungal infections, athlete's foot, or ringworm. Store any unused salve in a cool, dark location.

AWESOME ADDITION Lavender and calendula have natural anti-inflammatory and antifungal properties, making them a great addition to any antifungal oil or salve. Steep 1 tablespoon of each herb in the coconut oil over low heat for 2 hours. Strain before using in this recipe.

LAVENDER ANTIFUNGAL FOOT BATH

MAKES 1 TREATMENT ❧ TOPICAL

	3–6 mo.	6–24 mo.	2–6 yr.	6+ yr.
Lavender essential oil	no drops	no drops	4 drops	6 drops
Aloe vera gel	2 tbsp.	2 tbsp.	2 tbsp.	2 tbsp.
Epsom salt	2 tbsp.	2 tbsp.	2 tbsp.	2 tbsp.
Baking soda	1 tbsp.	1 tbsp.	1 tbsp.	1 tbsp.
Hot water	to fill	to fill	to fill	to fill

1. In a small bowl, stir together the lavender essential oil and aloe vera gel.
2. Place the Epsom salt and baking soda in a small bowl and stir in the aloe vera mixture
3. Pour the mixture into a large bucket or bowl and fill the bucket with hot water.
4. Have your child soak their feet in the foot bath for at least 20 minutes.

AWESOME ADDITION Soothing antifungal herbs such as lavender and calendula make great additions to this foot bath. Steep ½ cup (total) of the herbs in boiling water for 15 to 20 minutes before using in this recipe.

Balanitis

Bacteria, fungi, and chemicals found in many diapers and laundry detergents are the main causes of *balanitis*—inflammation of the penis head. Although balanitis mostly affects uncircumcised boys, circumcised boys may develop it as well. Anti-inflammatory and skin-healing essential oils such as lavender, tea tree, geranium, chamomile, and palmarosa help soothe inflammation and heal the skin.

CLEANSING ANTI-INFLAMMATORY SITZ BATH
MAKES 1 TREATMENT ❧ TOPICAL

	3–6 mo.	6–24 mo.	2–6 yr.	6+ yr.
German chamomile essential oil	no drops	1 drop	1 drop	2 drops
Lavender essential oil	2 drops	3 drops	4 drops	4 drops
Palmarosa essential oil	no drops	1 drop	1 drop	2 drops
Aloe vera gel	¼ cup	¼ cup	¼ cup	¼ cup
Epsom salt	1 cup	1 cup	1 cup	1 cup

1. In a small bowl, stir together the German chamomile, lavender, and palmarosa essential oils with the aloe vera gel.
2. Place the Epsom salt in a medium bowl and stir in the aloe vera mixture.
3. Pour the mixture under the running bath water, filling the tub quarter to half full.
4. Have your child sit in the bath and soak the bottom half of their body for at least 20 minutes.

HEALING BALANITIS SALVE

MAKES ABOUT 4 OUNCES ⇒ TOPICAL

	3–6 mo.	6–24 mo.	2–6 yr.	6+ yr.
Unrefined coconut oil	¼ cup	¼ cup	¼ cup	¼ cup
Beeswax pastilles	2 tbsp.	2 tbsp.	2 tbsp.	2 tbsp.
Unrefined shea butter	2 tbsp.	2 tbsp.	2 tbsp.	2 tbsp.
Geranium essential oil	no drops	5 drops	6 drops	10 drops
German chamomile essential oil	2 drops	5 drops	10 drops	20 drops
Tea tree essential oil	2 drops	10 drops	20 drops	50 drops

1. In a small pan over low heat, melt the coconut oil, beeswax, and shea butter.
2. Once melted, remove from heat, and add the geranium, German chamomile, and tea tree essential oils.
3. Pour into a Mason jar, and put into the freezer for 20 minutes to harden.
4. Cleanse and pat dry the affected areas, then apply the salve. Store any unused salve in a cool, dark location.

AWESOME ADDITION Lavender and calendula are well known for their anti-inflammatory and skin-healing properties. Steep ¼ cup (total) of the herbs in the coconut oil over low heat for 2 hours. Strain before using in this recipe.

Bedtime Fears

Bedtime fears can happen at any age. When my son became irrationally scared of monsters in his closet after moving into a new home, I created my Monsters-B-Gone blend to help him. I had him watch me overdramatically create this blend like a mad scientist in her laboratory and gave him the bottle to spray away his fears in all corners of his bedroom and closet. That night he slept until morning, with no middle-of-the-night wakeups. We haven't had anymore bedtime fears since then. This blend smells so good, it doubles as a great calming bedtime blend in the diffuser.

MONSTERS-B-GONE AROMATHERAPY ROOM SPRAY
MAKES 4 OUNCES ❧ AROMATIC

	3–6 mo.	6–24 mo.	2–6 yr.	6+ yr.
Filtered water	5 oz.	5 oz.	5 oz.	5 oz.
Witch hazel	2 tbsp.	2 tbsp.	2 tbsp.	2 tbsp.
Lavender essential oil	5 drops	10 drops	20 drops	40 drops
Roman chamomile essential oil	2 drops	4 drops	8 drops	16 drops
Tangerine essential oil	3 drops	6 drops	12 drops	24 drops
Vanilla CO_2 (12%)	2 drops	4 drops	8 drops	16 drops

1. Add ingredients to a spray bottle and shake to combine.
2. Spray around the room and on pillows and furniture.

SAFETY TIP Avoid spraying directly into the face. Spray away from the body.

MONSTERS-B-GONE DIFFUSER BLEND

MAKES ½ OUNCE ❧ AROMATIC

1½ teaspoons lavender essential oil
1 teaspoon tangerine essential oil

½ teaspoon Roman chamomile essential oil
25 drops vanilla CO_2 (12%)

TO MAKE THE BLEND

Add all the essential oils to an empty essential oil bottle (or any dark glass bottle with a dropper) and gently swirl the bottle to combine.

TO DIFFUSE THE BLEND

Add the recommended drops to a diffuser and diffuse throughout the room in 30-minute increments (30 minutes on/30 minutes off).

0–6 mo.	6–24 mo.	2–6 yr.	6+ yr.
2 drops	4 drops	6 drops	8 drops

Blisters

Blisters, especially when on your feet, can be very painful. Most doctors agree that allowing blisters to air out, removing bandages if there are any, and giving them a chance to breathe and dry out helps them heal faster. Antibacterial and skin-healing essential oils such as lavender, tea tree, palmarosa, rosalina, marjoram, geranium, neroli, petitgrain, chamomile, fir needle, cypress, cedarwood, sweet orange, lemon, and blue tansy can help soothe the pain and heal blisters faster without infection.

HEALING BLISTER SPRAY

MAKES ABOUT 4 OUNCES ⋙ TOPICAL

	3–6 mo.	6–24 mo.	2–6 yr.	6+ yr.
Witch hazel	2 tbsp.	2 tbsp.	2 tbsp.	2 tbsp.
Aloe vera gel	1½ tsp.	1½ tsp.	1½ tsp.	1½ tsp.
Vegetable glycerin	½ tsp.	½ tsp.	½ tsp.	½ tsp.
Lavender essential oil	1 drop	2 drops	4 drops	8 drops
Tea tree essential oil	1 drop	2 drops	4 drops	8 drops
Filtered water	to fill	to fill	to fill	to fill

1. Combine the witch hazel, aloe vera gel, vegetable glycerin, and the lavender and tea tree essential oils in a 4-ounce spray bottle. Gently swirl the bottle to combine.

2. Add enough filtered water to fill the bottle.

3. To use, spray onto blisters and gently pat dry with a clean cloth or towel. Follow with Anti-Blister Salve (page 127). Store any unused spray in a cool, dark location.

SUBSTITUTION TIP For extra skin-healing benefits, substitute calendula or chamomile hydrosol with the water in this recipe. Both chamomile and calendula are well known for their abilities to soothe inflammation, boost tissue regeneration, and heal wounds.

ANTI-BLISTER SALVE
MAKES ABOUT 4 OUNCES ❧ TOPICAL

	3–6 mo.	6–24 mo.	2–6 yr.	6+ yr.
Unrefined coconut oil	¼ cup	¼ cup	¼ cup	¼ cup
Beeswax pastilles	2 tbsp.	2 tbsp.	2 tbsp.	2 tbsp.
Shea butter	2 tbsp.	2 tbsp.	2 tbsp.	2 tbsp.
Geranium essential oil	no drops	5 drops	10 drops	15 drops
Lavender essential oil	4 drops	10 drops	20 drops	40 drops
Tea tree essential oil	no drops	5 drops	10 drops	20 drops

1. In a small pan over low heat, combine the coconut oil, beeswax, and shea butter.
2. Once melted, remove from heat, and add the geranium, lavender, and tea tree essential oils.
3. Pour into a Mason jar, and put into the freezer for 20 minutes to harden.
4. Apply the salve to clean blisters as needed. Store any unused salve in a cool, dark location.

AWESOME ADDITION Calendula is well known for its anti-inflammatory and skin-healing properties. It would make a great addition to this salve. Steep ¼ cup of the herb in the coconut oil over low heat for 2 hours. Strain before using in this recipe.

HEALING BLISTER FOOT BATH

MAKES 1 TREATMENT ⚬ TOPICAL

	3–6 mo.	6–24 mo.	2–6 yr.	6+ yr.
Lavender essential oil	no drops	no drops	4 drops	6 drops
Palmarosa essential oil	no drops	no drops	2 drops	2 drops
Aloe vera gel	2 tbsp.	2 tbsp.	2 tbsp.	2 tbsp.
Epsom salt	½ cup	½ cup	½ cup	½ cup
Hot water	to fill	to fill	to fill	to fill

1. In a small bowl, stir together the lavender and palmarosa essential oils with the aloe vera gel.
2. Place the Epsom salt in a medium bowl and stir in the aloe vera mixture.
3. Pour the mixture into a large bucket or bowl and fill with hot water (enough to cover the feet and ankles).
4. Have your child soak their feet in the bath for at least 20 minutes.

Bronchitis

A complication of a viral or bacterial infection, bronchitis starts with cold- or flu-like symptoms—runny nose, dry cough, and even sore throat. As the infection progresses, the bronchial tubes become inflamed. Symptoms of bronchitis include a dry painful cough, fever, yellow-colored phlegm, chest pain, and wheezing. Aromatherapy is specially suited to treating lung infections and can help soothe the cough, expel phlegm, and help the body fight off the infection faster. Anti-inflammatory and expectorant essential oils that help open up the airways include lavender, rosalina, fir needle, tea tree, palmarosa, cypress, pine, marjoram, chamomile, spearmint, frankincense, petitgrain, spruce, sandalwood, and ginger.

BREATHE BETTER BRONCHITIS DIFFUSER BLEND
MAKES ½ OUNCE ❧ AROMATIC

1 teaspoon fir needle essential oil
1 teaspoon rosalina essential oil

½ teaspoon cypress essential oil
½ teaspoon lavender essential oil

TO MAKE THE BLEND

Add all the essential oils to an empty essential oil bottle (or any dark glass bottle with a dropper), and gently swirl the bottle to combine.

TO DIFFUSE THE BLEND

Add the recommended drops to a diffuser and diffuse throughout the room in 30-minute increments (30 minutes on/30 minutes off).

0–6 mo.	6–24 mo.	2–6 yr.	6+ yr.
2 drops	4 drops	6 drops	8 drops

BRONCHIAL CHEST RUB
MAKES ABOUT 4 OUNCES ❧ AROMATIC ❧ TOPICAL

	3–6 mo.	6–24 mo.	2–6 yr.	6+ yr.
Unrefined coconut oil	½ cup	½ cup	½ cup	½ cup
Fir needle essential oil	1 drop	4 drops	8 drops	20 drops
Lavender essential oil	1 drop	4 drops	8 drops	20 drops
Rosalina essential oil	2 drops	8 drops	16 drops	30 drops

1. In a small pan over low heat, melt the coconut oil.
2. Once melted, remove from heat, add the fir needle, lavender, and rosalina essential oils, and stir to combine. ➤

3. Pour into a Mason jar, and put into the freezer for 20 minutes, to harden.
4. Rub onto your baby's chest, back, and the bottoms of their feet. Cover the feet with socks. Store any unused rub in a cool, dark location.

SAFETY TIP Do not apply chest rub to your child's face or under their nose.

BRONCHITIS BUSTER AROMATHERAPY SHOWER STEAMERS
MAKES 12 SHOWER STEAMERS ✣ AROMATIC

	3–6 mo.	6–24 mo.	2–6 yr.	6+ yr.
Baking soda	1 cup	1 cup	1 cup	1 cup
Arrowroot powder or cornstarch	⅓ cup	⅓ cup	⅓ cup	⅓ cup
Water	⅓ cup + 2 tbsp.	⅓ cup + 2 tbsp.	⅓ cup + 2 tbsp.	⅓ cup + 2 tbsp.
Fir needle essential oil	1 drop	2 drops	2 drops	2 drops
Frankincense essential oil	no drops	1 drop	1 drop	1 drop
Rosalina essential oil	2 drops	2 drops	2 drops	2 drops

1. Preheat oven to 350°F.
2. In a medium bowl, combine the baking soda, arrowroot powder, and water to make a thick paste.
3. Pour the mixture into a 12-cup silicone muffin pan, filling each cup halfway.
4. Bake in the oven for 20 minutes. Allow to sit out overnight if extra dry time is needed.
5. Pop out of the molds and store the discs in a wide-mouthed Mason jar.
6. To use, add the essential oils to one disc, then place it at the far side of the shower, away from the water. Close the bathroom door and breathe in.

Bug Bites and Stings

Bug bites and stings can cause a variety of reactions depending on the allergies of the person, what type of bug did the biting or stinging, and how many bites or stings were acquired. If you or your child is bitten by a suspected poisonous snake or arachnid, seek medical attention immediately. Antibacterial and anti-inflammatory essential oils soothe the itch, reduce inflammation, and heal up any wounds from minor bites and stings. Try lavender, tea tree, rosalina, geranium, chamomile, blue tansy, frankincense, spearmint, palmarosa, fir needle, cypress, juniper berry, pine, neroli, coriander, patchouli, marjoram, rose, and sandalwood.

SOOTHE THE STING BEE STING ROLL-ON RELIEF
MAKES ⅓ OUNCE ⇒ SAFE FOR AGES 3+ MONTHS ⇒ TOPICAL

⅛ teaspoon baking soda

¼ teaspoon liquid castile soap

2 drops lavender essential oil

Filtered water, to fill

1. In a ⅓-ounce glass roll-on bottle, combine the baking soda, liquid castile soap, and lavender essential oil.

2. Add enough filtered water to fill the bottle. Place the roller ball and cap on and shake well to blend. Don't forget to label your creation.

3. To apply, remove the stinger completely from the wound. Shake the remedy well. Roll on to soothe, applying up to 5 times a day until the swelling is completely gone.

4. Follow with a treatment of Healing Antiseptic Boo-Boo Balm (page 161) until the wound is completely healed.

HELPFUL HINT Bee and wasp stings do not have the same type of venom and need different remedies to soothe their sting. Bee venom is naturally acidic, so a natural remedy using more alkaline ingredients (including baking soda and castile soap) can help to neutralize the sting.

ANTI-ITCH CALAMINE LOTION

MAKES ABOUT 4 OUNCES ❧ TOPICAL

	3–6 mo.	6–24 mo.	2–6 yr.	6+ yr.
Bentonite clay	3 tbsp.	3 tbsp.	3 tbsp.	3 tbsp.
Baking soda	2 tbsp.	2 tbsp.	2 tbsp.	2 tbsp.
Vegetable glycerin	1 tbsp.	1 tbsp.	1 tbsp.	1 tbsp.
Lavender essential oil	3 drops	15 drops	15 drops	15 drops
Tea tree essential oil	1 drop	5 drops	5 drops	5 drops
Filtered water or witch hazel	enough to form a paste	enough to form a paste	enough to form a paste	enough to form a paste

1. Add the baking soda, clay, vegetable glycerin, and essential oils to a Mason jar, and stir to combine.
2. Add the filtered water 1 tablespoon at a time, stirring after each addition, to form a paste-like consistency.
3. Apply to itchy bug bites, rashes, and burns to relieve itchiness, pain, and inflammation.
4. Cover and store in the refrigerator when not in use.

SOOTHE THE STING WASP STING ROLL-ON RELIEF

MAKES ⅓ OUNCE ⇝ SAFE FOR AGES 3+ MONTHS ⇝ TOPICAL

¼ teaspoon raw unfiltered apple
   cider vinegar
¼ teaspoon aloe vera gel

2 drops lavender essential oil
Filtered water, to fill

1. In a ⅓-ounce roll-on bottle, combine the apple cider vinegar, aloe vera gel, and lavender essential oil.

2. Add enough filtered water to fill the bottle. Place the roller ball and cap on and shake well to blend. Don't forget to label your creation.

3. To apply, remove the stinger completely from the wound. Shake the remedy well. Roll on to soothe, applying up to 5 times a day until the swelling is completely gone.

4. Follow with a treatment of Healing Antiseptic Boo Boo Balm (page 161) until the wound is completely healed.

HELPFUL HINT Bee stings and wasp stings do not have the same type of venom and need different remedies to soothe their stings. Wasp sting venom is naturally alkaline, so a natural remedy using more acidic ingredients, including apple cider vinegar and aloe vera gel, can help to neutralize the sting.

Bug Repellents

Not all bug repellents are alike. If you are trying to avoid toxic bug repellents containing dangerous pesticides like DEET, many essential oils have repelling and killing properties to them. Citronella essential oil is one of the most commonly used bug-repelling essential oils. It repels most bugs and arachnids and smells amazing. Cedarwood essential oil is one of my favorite bug repelling essential oils. When combined with sweet orange essential oil, it can repel and kill any bug in the vicinity of your spraying. Other essential oils that repel bugs include lavender, spearmint, rosalina, lemon, patchouli, geranium, grapefruit, lemon, tangerine, mandarin, pine, and tea tree.

BUGS-B-GONE JR. BODY SPRAY

MAKES ABOUT 4 OUNCES ❧ TOPICAL

	3–6 mo.	6–24 mo.	2–6 yr.	6+ yr.
Witch hazel	2 tbsp.	2 tbsp.	2 tbsp.	2 tbsp.
Aloe vera gel	1 tbsp.	1 tbsp.	1 tbsp.	1 tbsp.
Vegetable glycerin	½ tsp.	½ tsp.	½ tsp.	½ tsp.
Atlas cedarwood essential oil	no drops	5 drops	10 drops	15 drops
Citronella essential oil	no drops	10 drops	20 drops	30 drops
Sweet orange essential oil	5 drops	5 drops	10 drops	15 drops
Filtered water	to fill	to fill	to fill	to fill

1. Combine the witch hazel, aloe vera gel, vegetable glycerin, and the Atlas cedarwood, citronella, and sweet orange essential oils in a 4-ounce spray bottle. Gently swirl the bottle to combine.

2. Add enough filtered water to fill the bottle.

3. Shake well before use. Spray onto your child's hair and body, avoiding the face. Store any unused spray in a cool, dark location.

BUGS-B-GONE JR. SALVE
MAKES ABOUT 4 OUNCES ❧ TOPICAL

	3–6 mo.	6–24 mo.	2–6 yr.	6+ yr.
Unrefined coconut oil	¼ cup	¼ cup	¼ cup	¼ cup
Beeswax pastilles	2 tbsp.	2 tbsp.	2 tbsp.	2 tbsp.
Extra-virgin olive oil	2 tbsp.	2 tbsp.	2 tbsp.	2 tbsp.
Atlas cedarwood essential oil	no drops	5 drops	10 drops	15 drops
Citronella essential oil	no drops	10 drops	20 drops	30 drops
Lavender essential oil	4 drops	5 drops	10 drops	15 drops

1. In a small pan over low heat, melt the coconut oil, beeswax, and olive oil.
2. Once melted, remove from heat, and add the Atlas cedarwood, citronella, and lavender essential oils.
3. Pour into a Mason jar, and put into the freezer for 20 minutes to harden.
4. Apply the salve all over your child's skin, avoiding the face. Store any unused salve in a cool, dark location.

BUGS-B-GONE JR. CITRONELLA CANDLES
MAKES ABOUT 8 OUNCES ❧ SAFE FOR ALL AGES ❧ AROMATIC

30 drops citronella essential oil
25 drops Atlas cedarwood essential oil
25 drops lemon eucalyptus essential oil

1. Place 1 soy wick in an empty Mason jar or recycled candle jar.
2. In a small pan over low heat, melt the soy wax. Once melted, remove from heat, and add the citronella, Atlas cedarwood, and lemon eucalyptus essential oils. Stir to combine. ➜

3. Pour the wax mixture into the prepared jar and allow to cool and harden at room temperature.

4. Bring the candles with you on your picnics and BBQs. Light the candles and let them repel the bugs while you enjoy your outdoor fun.

HELPFUL HINT To keep the wick in place while the candle cools, lay two chopsticks or butter knives flat across the top of the jar, parallel to each other, with the wick in the middle. This will help keep the wick from falling to the sides while the wax hardens.

Burns and Sunburns

Hot objects, hot liquids, steam, electricity, radiation, the sun, and even chemicals—no matter our vigilance, sometimes accident occur. It's very important to assess burns for severity before deciding on the best course of action. Electrical burns are often worse than they look, so immediate medical attention is required. If a burn is more than just superficial (second- or third-degree), seek immediate medical attention.

No matter the severity of a burn, immediately cool it by submerging the area in cold water, but do not use ice. Treating the burn with gently running water for 10 minutes or submerging it in a bowl or sink works well. Don't apply oils, butters, or salves to burned areas until completely cooled. After Sun Spray (page 138) can help cool down affected areas before applying either Soothing Burn Oil (below) or After Sun Salve (page 137) to cleaned, dried burns.

SOOTHING BURN OIL
MAKES ABOUT 2 OUNCES ✴ TOPICAL

	3–6 mo.	6–24 mo.	2–6 yr.	6+ yr.
Unrefined coconut oil	¼ cup	¼ cup	¼ cup	¼ cup
Lavender essential oil	2 drops	9 drops	18 drops	20 drops
Vitamin E oil (optional)	1 tsp.	1 tsp.	1 tsp.	1 tsp.

1. In a pan over low heat, melt the coconut oil.
2. Once melted, remove from heat, and add the lavender essential oil and vitamin E oil (if using).
3. Pour into a Mason jar, and put into the freezer for 20 minutes to harden.
4. Apply a small amount as needed to clean, dry burns.

SAFETY TIP Do not use essential oils with children under 3 months old. Simply omit from this recipe. You could also infuse the herb of lavender into the coconut oil, for a gentler option.

AFTER SUN SALVE
MAKES ABOUT 4 OUNCES ≫ TOPICAL

	3–6 mo.	6–24 mo.	2–6 yr.	6+ yr.
Unrefined coconut oil	¼ cup	¼ cup	¼ cup	¼ cup
Beeswax	2 tbsp.	2 tbsp.	2 tbsp.	2 tbsp.
Unrefined shea butter	2 tbsp.	2 tbsp.	2 tbsp.	2 tbsp.
Rosalina essential oil	2 drops	8 drops	15 drops	15 drops
Lavender essential oil	2 drops	10 drops	20 drops	15 drops
Vitamin E oil (optional)	1 tsp.	1 tsp.	1 tsp.	1 tsp.

1. In a pan over low heat, melt the coconut oil, beeswax, and shea butter.
2. Once melted, remove from heat, and add the lavender and rosalina essential oils, and the vitamin E oil (if using).
3. Pour into a 4-ounce Mason jar, and put into the freezer for 20 minutes to harden.
4. Apply a small amount as needed to clean, dry burns.

SAFETY TIP Do not use essential oils with children under 3 months old. Simply omit from this recipe. You could also infuse the lavender buds into the coconut oil, for a gentler option.

AFTER SUN SPRAY

MAKES ABOUT 8 OUNCES ≫ TOPICAL

	3–6 mo.	6–24 mo.	2–6 yr.	6+ yr.
Peppermint hydrosol	¼ cup + 2 tbsp.	¼ cup + 2 tbsp.	¼ cup + 2 tbsp.	¼ cup + 2 tbsp.
Aloe vera gel	¼ cup	¼ cup	¼ cup	¼ cup
Raw unfiltered apple cider vinegar	1 tbsp.	1 tbsp.	1 tbsp.	1 tbsp.
German chamomile essential oil	2 drops	3 drops	5 drops	5 drops
Lavender essential oil	4 drops	7 drops	10 drops	10 drops
Filtered water	to fill	to fill	to fill	to fill

1. Add the peppermint hydrosol, aloe vera gel, apple cider vinegar, and the German chamomile and lavender essential oils to an 8-ounce spray bottle.

2. Add enough filtered water to fill, and gently swirl to combine.

3. Shake well before use. Spray onto burns as often as needed for pain relief, or at least once daily to help heal the burn faster. Once the skin is cooled from the initial burn, follow up with a healing burn salve to keep the skin moisturized while it heals. Keep in the refrigerator for extra cooling and a longer shelf life (6 to 9 months).

HELPFUL HINT This spray can help on burns in the kitchen, too. I like to keep this spray in my refrigerator when not in use because the cool temperature is very soothing on fresh burns and can help relieve some of the pain. Remember to shake well before use.

Catarrh

When fighting a virus or bacteria, one of the human body's amazing self-defense mechanisms is to produce phlegm. Producing too much mucus in the throat and nose is called *catarrh*. Catarrh can be treated with breathing treatments containing lavender, rosalina, fir needle, tea tree, palmarosa, cypress, pine, marjoram, chamomile, spearmint, frankincense, petitgrain, spruce, sandalwood, and ginger, and chest rubs containing expectorant and anti-inflammatory essential oils including lavender, rosalina, fir needle, tea tree, palmarosa, cypress, pine, marjoram, chamomile, spearmint, frankincense, petitgrain, spruce, sandalwood, and ginger.

EXPECTORANT HUMIDIFIER BLEND

MAKES ½ OUNCE ❧ AROMATIC

1 teaspoon marjoram essential oil
1 teaspoon rosalina essential oil
½ teaspoon lavender essential oil

½ teaspoon Roman chamomile
essential oil

TO MAKE THE BLEND

Add all the essential oils to an empty essential oil bottle (or any dark glass bottle with a dropper), and gently swirl the bottle to combine.

TO DIFFUSE THE BLEND

Add the recommended drops to a diffuser and diffuse throughout the room in 30-minute increments (30 minutes on/30 minutes off).

0–6 mo.	6–24 mo.	2–6 yr.	6+ yr.
2 drops	4 drops	6 drops	8 drops

MUCUS MONSTER HERBAL SALT STEAM

MAKES 1 TREATMENT ⚬ AROMATIC

	3–6 mo.	6–24 mo.	2–6 yr.	6+ yr.
Frankincense essential oil	no drops	1 drop	2 drops	2 drops
Lavender essential oil	2 drops	2 drops	2 drops	2 drops
Rosalina essential oil	2 drops	2 drops	3 drops	3 drops
Sea salt	¼ cup	¼ cup	¼ cup	¼ cup

1. In a small bowl, mix the frankincense, lavender, and rosalina essential oils with the sea salt until distributed evenly. Transfer the mixture to a large bowl.
2. Bring 4 to 6 cups of water to a boil. Pour the boiling water over the salt mixture and stir to combine.
3. For children 6 years and older, cover their head with a towel and position their face over the bowl, using the towel as a tent to hold the steam in. Let them sit with their eyes closed, over the steam, breathing the steam for no more than 10 minutes at a time.
4. For babies and children younger than 6 years, make a "tent" with a blanket or sheet and sit with them around the bowl.

AWESOME ADDITION Herbal steams have been used for centuries to heal chest infections. Lavender, rosemary, sage, and thyme are all great additions to this steam. Add ¼ cup (total) of the herbs to a cloth tea bag or an old, clean sock, and steep in the boiling water for 15 to 20 minutes before using the steam.

EXPECTORANT CHEST RUB

MAKES ABOUT 4 OUNCES ≫ TOPICAL ≫ AROMATIC

	3–6 mo.	6–24 mo.	2–6 yr.	6+ yr.
Unrefined coconut oil	½ cup	½ cup	½ cup	½ cup
Fir needle essential oil	2 drops	10 drops	15 drops	20 drops
Lavender essential oil	2 drops	5 drops	10 drops	10 drops
Marjoram essential oil	no drops	5 drops	10 drops	15 drops

1. In a small pan over low heat, melt the coconut oil.
2. Once melted, remove from heat and add the essential oils.
3. Pour into a Mason jar, and put into the freezer for 20 minutes to harden.
4. Rub onto your baby's chest, back, and the bottoms of their feet. Cover their feet with socks. Store any unused rub in a cool, dark location.

SAFETY TIP Do not apply chest rub to a child's face or under their nose.

Chicken Pox

Caused by a viral infection, chicken pox can only be contracted by direct contact with another person who has chicken pox or shingles. It is very contagious, and while it's usually safe in childhood, it can be dangerous for those who contract it for the first time in adulthood. Essential oils can be used to calm the itch, heal the sores, and even kill the highly contagious germs in the air. Antiviral and soothing skin-healing essential oils including lavender, tea tree, marjoram, rosalina, neroli, spearmint, lemon, sweet orange, frankincense, coriander, petitgrain, geranium, rose, and palmarosa can help.

SOOTHING ANTI-ITCH OAT BATH

MAKES 1 TREATMENT ⇒ TOPICAL

	3–6 mo.	6–24 mo.	2–6 yr.	6+ yr.
Oats, finely ground	1 cup	1 cup	1 cup	1 cup
Baking soda	¼ cup	¼ cup	¼ cup	¼ cup
German chamomile essential oil	1 drop	1 drop	3 drops	3 drops
Lavender essential oil	1 drop	2 drops	3 drops	4 drops

1. Pulse the oats in a blender or food processor until powdered. Add the baking soda and pulse until well mixed.
2. Add the German chamomile and lavender essential oil drops and pulse a few times more to mix them in.
3. To use, either add straight to the bath under running water or add to a fine mesh bag or an old, clean sock, tie closed and toss into the bathtub under the running water. Have your child soak in the tub at least 20 minutes. Store any unused bath mix in a Mason jar in a cool dry location.

HELPFUL HINT To keep skin moisturized, do not wipe skin dry when getting out of the tub. Gently pat it dry instead and follow with a treatment of Ultra Moisturizing Body Butter (page 169) or Anti-Itch Calamine Lotion (below).

ANTI-ITCH CALAMINE LOTION

MAKES ABOUT 4 OUNCES ⇒ TOPICAL

	3–6 mo.	6–24 mo.	2–6 yr.	6+ yr.
Lavender essential oil	3 drops	15 drops	15 drops	15 drops
Rosalina essential oil	1 drop	5 drops	5 drops	5 drops

1. Add the essential oils to a Mason jar and stir to combine.
2. Apply the lotion to itchy sores as often as needed to relieve itchiness, pain, and inflammation. Store any unused lotion in the refrigerator.

KILL THE GERMS ANTIVIRAL DIFFUSER BLEND
MAKES ½ OUNCE ❧ AROMATIC ❧ PHOTOSENSITIZING

1 teaspoon lemon essential oil
¾ teaspoon coriander essential oil

¾ teaspoon lavender essential oil
½ teaspoon rosalina essential oil

TO MAKE THE BLEND
Add all the essential oils to an empty essential oil bottle (or any dark glass bottle with a dropper), and gently swirl the bottle to combine.

TO DIFFUSE THE BLEND
Add the recommended drops to a diffuser and diffuse throughout the room in 30-minute increments (30 minutes on/30 minutes off).

0–6 mo.	6–24 mo.	2–6 yr.	6+ yr.
2 drops	4 drops	6 drops	8 drops

HELPFUL HINT This essential oil blend can be used diluted in coconut oil or aloe vera gel as an antiviral hand sanitizer. This blend is strong, and contains photosensitizing lemon oil, so don't forget to dilute before using topically, and use caution in the sun.

Circumcision

If you have chosen to get your son circumcised, special care should be taken during the recovery period. It can take 7 to 10 days to heal from a circumcision, though most procedures done now are so simple that if you take proper care, he can heal up in a couple of days. Essential oils are not recommended for babies under 3 months old because of their thin, sensitive skin, but hydrosols are the perfect gentle option to cleanse the incision, reduce inflammation, and help the wound site heal up in record time.

ANTIBACTERIAL CLEANSING CIRCUMCISION WASH

MAKES ABOUT 4 OUNCES ❧ SAFE FOR ALL AGES ❧ TOPICAL

¼ cup lavender hydrosol
1 tablespoon aloe vera gel
1 teaspoon vegetable glycerin

2 tablespoons witch hazel
Filtered water, to fill

1. Add the lavender hydrosol, vegetable glycerin, aloe vera gel, and witch hazel to a 4-ounce spray bottle. Gently swirl the bottle to combine.
2. Add enough filtered water to fill the bottle.
3. To use, after each diaper change, spray onto the penis and gently pat dry with a clean cloth or towel. Follow with Simple Healing Lavender Salve (below). Store any unused wash in a cool, dark location.

SOOTHING LAVENDER CIRCUMCISION COMPRESS

MAKES 1 TREATMENT ❧ SAFE FOR ALL AGES ❧ TOPICAL

½ cup lavender hydrosol
2 tablespoons aloe vera gel

1 tablespoon sea salt
Warm water

1. In a medium bowl, combine the lavender hydrosol, aloe vera gel, and sea salt.
2. Stir in enough warm water to fill the bowl most of the way, leaving room to dip the washcloth.
3. To use, dip a washcloth into the mixture and squeeze out any excess. Gently apply to the penis for 5 minutes at a time. The compress can be used as often as needed to reduce inflammation, redness, and pain.

SIMPLE HEALING LAVENDER SALVE

MAKES 4 OUNCES ❧ SAFE FOR ALL AGES ❧ TOPICAL

¼ cup unrefined coconut oil
2 tablespoons lavender buds

2 tablespoons beeswax pastilles
2 tablespoons unrefined shea butter

1. In a small pan over low heat, melt the coconut oil.
2. Add the lavender buds and steep for 1 hour. Strain with a fine mesh strainer.
3. Add the beeswax and shea butter to the strained oil and melt over low heat.

4. Once melted, remove from heat, and pour into a Mason jar. Put into the freezer for 20 minutes to harden.

5. Apply the salve to the penis head after gently cleansing with the Anti-bacterial Cleansing Circumcision Wash (page 144) and patting dry. Store the salve in a cool, dark location.

Colds

Characterized by a stuffy, runny nose, sore throat, cough, congestion, and even sometimes a fever, colds are different for everyone. Diffusion of antibacterial and antiviral essential oils such as lavender, tea tree, lemon, cinnamon, frankincense, marjoram, rosalina, cypress, palmarosa, spearmint, and fir needle can help cleanse the air of germs. Topically, essential oils can help calm a cough, cool a fever, and even boost the immune system to beat the cold faster.

JUNIOR DIFFUSER BLEND
MAKES ½ OUNCE ⤳ AROMATIC

1 teaspoon fir needle essential oil

¾ teaspoon cinnamon leaf essential oil

¾ teaspoon lavender essential oil

½ teaspoon frankincense essential oil

TO MAKE THE BLEND

Add all the essential oils to an empty essential oil bottle (or any dark glass bottle with a dropper) and gently swirl the bottle to combine.

TO DIFFUSE THE BLEND

Add the recommended drops to a diffuser and diffuse throughout the room in 30-minute increments (30 minutes on/30 minutes off).

0–6 mo.	6–24 mo.	2–6 yr.	6+ yr.
2 drops	4 drops	6 drops	8 drops

SAFETY TIP Cinnamon bark essential oil is too harsh for topical application but is perfectly safe to use in diffusion. Cinnamon leaf essential oil is much gentler, however, and can be used in both diffusion and at a low dilution in topical applications.

FEEL BETTER BATH

MAKES 1 TREATMENT ⇝ TOPICAL ⇝ AROMATIC

	3–6 mo.	6–24 mo.	2–6 yr.	6+ yr.
Lavender essential oil	1 drop	1 drop	1 drop	2 drops
Marjoram essential oil	no drops	1 drop	2 drops	3 drops
Rosalina essential oil	1 drop	2 drops	3 drops	3 drops
Unscented liquid castile soap or baby shampoo	1 tbsp.	1 tbsp.	1 tbsp.	1 tbsp.
Epsom salt	1 cup	1 cup	1 cup	1 cup

1. In a small bowl, stir together the lavender, marjoram, and rosalina essential oils with the castile soap.

2. Place the Epsom salt in a medium bowl and stir in the soap mixture.

3. Pour the mixture under the running bath water as you fill the tub.

AWESOME ADDITION Soothing antibacterial and immune supporting herbs such as lavender and calendula make great additions to this bath. Add ¼ cup of each herb to a cloth tea bag or an old, clean sock, and tie closed before tossing into the bathtub.

GERM-KILLER FOAMING HAND SOAP

MAKES 8 OUNCES ➣ SAFE FOR AGES 3+ MONTHS ➣ TOPICAL

1 tablespoon liquid castile soap
1 tablespoon vegetable glycerin
5 drops lavender essential oil

3 drops rosalina essential oil
Filtered water, to fill

1. Combine the castile soap, vegetable glycerin, and the lavender and rosalina essential oils in a foaming handsoap bottle. Gently swirl the bottle to combine.

2. Add enough filtered water to fill the bottle. Shake well to combine. Wash hands often to kill germs.

SUBSTITUTION TIP For extra-gentle antibacterial benefits, substitute lavender hydrosol for the water in this recipe. Lavender is well known for its abilities to soothe inflammation, cleanse a wound, and heal dry skin.

Cold Sores (Fever Blisters)

Cold sores, small blisters that pop up around or inside the mouth, on the lips, and even in the throat, are a symptom of the herpes simplex 1 virus (HSV-1). This virus is extremely contagious and is spread through kissing, sharing utensils, and sharing cups. Once infected with the herpes virus, a person has it for life, getting periodic breakouts in the same spots. Breakouts can occur when stressed, in the presence of other viruses such as the flu, or if the weather is hot. Unfortunately, like most viruses, herpes doesn't discriminate. It's estimated 1 in 5 Americans has HSV-1, and some of those people are children. This can be very scary for parents, but it's good to know that you can help alleviate some of the pain, and prevent future breakouts with natural remedies. Antiviral essential oils such as lavender, geranium, lemon, chamomile, spearmint, coriander, rosalina, and tea tree all help reduce the occurrence of cold sores if used at the first tingling signs of an outbreak.

COLD SORE SPOT TREATMENT

MAKES ABOUT 1 OUNCE ❧ TOPICAL

	3–6 mo.	6–24 mo.	2–6 yr.	6+ yr.
Unrefined coconut oil	1 tbsp.	1 tbsp.	1 tbsp.	1 tbsp.
Vitamin E oil	1 tbsp.	1 tbsp.	1 tbsp.	1 tbsp.
German chamomile essential oil	1 drop	2 drops	3 drops	9 drops
Lavender essential oil	1 drop	2 drops	3 drops	9 drops

1. In a small pan over low heat, melt the coconut oil.
2. Once melted, remove from heat, and whisk in the vitamin E oil and the German chamomile and lavender essential oils.
3. Pour into a Mason jar, and put into the freezer for 20 minutes to harden.
4. Using a fresh cotton swab, apply a small amount of oil to each sore at the first signs of tingling. Store any unused oil in a cool, dark location.

COLD SORE RELIEF HEALING LIP BALM

MAKES ABOUT 3 OUNCES ❧ TOPICAL

	3–6 mo.	6–24 mo.	2–6 yr.	6+ yr.
Unrefined coconut oil	3 tbsp.	3 tbsp.	3 tbsp.	3 tbsp.
Beeswax pastilles	2 tbsp.	2 tbsp.	2 tbsp.	2 tbsp.
Shea butter	1 tbsp.	1 tbsp.	1 tbsp.	1 tbsp.
Vitamin E oil	1 tsp.	1 tsp.	1 tsp.	1 tsp.
Lavender essential oil	3 drops	6 drops	10 drops	15 drops
Lemon essential oil	no drops	3 drops	5 drops	10 drops

1. In a small pan over low heat, melt the coconut oil, beeswax, and shea butter.

2. Once melted, remove from heat and add the vitamin E oil and the lavender and lemon essential oils.

3. Pour into lip balm containers, tins, or jars.

4. Using a fresh cotton swab, apply a small amount of lip balm to your child's lips. Store any unused lip balm in a cool, dark location.

AWESOME ADDITION Lemon balm is well known for its antiviral and anti-inflammatory properties and is the most widely used herb in the treatment of cold sores. Steep 2 tablespoons of lemon balm in the coconut oil over low heat for 2 hours. Strain and continue with the recipe.

Colic

Colic is a common condition in infants that causes pain and discomfort in the abdomen area. Babies with colic will cry for hours on end, drawing their legs up to their stomach and clenching their fists. The cause of colic, which lasts from three to six weeks and usually disappears around the three-month-old mark, is still somewhat of a mystery. Thankfully, there are natural remedies that can help soothe and ease the pain for your baby. To soothe a colicky baby not yet old enough to use essential oils, hydrosols are the safest option.

COLIC BABY AROMATHERAPY ROLL-ON
MAKES ⅓ OUNCE ⪼ SAFE FOR ALL AGES ⪼ TOPICAL

Roman chamomile hydrosol

1. Fill a ⅓-ounce roll-on bottle with chamomile hydrosol. Place the roller ball and cap on and label your creation.

2. To use, roll onto your baby's abdomen, back, and chest. Gently massage into the skin.

CALM THE COLIC MAGNESIUM OIL SPRAY

MAKES 4 OUNCES ≫ SAFE FOR ALL AGES ≫ TOPICAL

½ cup lavender or Roman
  chamomile hydrosol

½ cup magnesium flakes

1. In a non-aluminum pan, bring the hydrosol to a boil.
2. Remove from heat and add the magnesium flakes, stirring until completely dissolved.
3. Pour into a 4-ounce spray bottle and store in a cool, dark location when not in use.
4. Spray onto your infant's abdomen and gently massage into the skin.

HELPFUL HINT This spray is not only great at calming colicky babies; it also soothes growing pains and lulls toddlers and children to sleep. Our bodies require magnesium to function, yet many of us are deficient in this mineral, including young children. Spray onto your child's body and massage into the skin as part of your bedtime routine. You can buy magnesium flakes online or at health and body stores.

COLIC CALMER BABY BATH

MAKES 1 TREATMENT ≫ SAFE FOR ALL AGES ≫ TOPICAL

1 cup Epsom salt

1 cup chamomile hydrosol

Pour both ingredients under the running bath water as you fill the tub.

AWESOME ADDITION Chamomile is a natural digestive and can help to calm and soothe a colicky baby. Add ½ cup of herb to a cloth tea bag or an old, clean sock, and tie closed before tossing into the bathtub.

Congestion

There are many causes to nasal and sinus congestion, including a cold, the flu, or allergies. The actual cause of nasal congestion is not too much mucus in the nasal passageways, but the inflammation of blood vessels in those passageways. When congested, keep the nasal passageways moist. Dry nasal passageways can irritate the mucous membranes and make congestion worse. A humidifier, saline nasal spray, and salt steams help relieve congestion and keep those membranes moist. Essential oils that help relieve inflammation and open up the airways include lavender, rosalina, fir needle, cypress, pine, juniper berry, lemon eucalyptus, spearmint, frankincense, spruce, lemon, cedarwood, and tea tree.

CLEAR THE CONGESTION SALT STEAM

MAKES 1 TREATMENT ≫ AROMATIC

	3–6 mo.	6–24 mo.	2–6 yr.	6+ yr.
Sea salt	¼ cup	¼ cup	¼ cup	¼ cup
Frankincense essential oil	no drops	1 drop	2 drops	2 drops
Lavender essential oil	1 drop	1 drop	2 drops	2 drops
Rosalina essential oil	1 drop	1 drop	2 drops	2 drops

1. In a small glass bowl, mix together the sea salt, and frankincense, lavender, and rosalina essential oils. Transfer to a large bowl.
2. Bring 4 to 6 cups of water to a boil. Pour the boiling water over the salt mixture.
3. For children 6 years and older, cover their head with a towel and position their face over the bowl, using the towel as a tent to hold the steam in. Let them sit with their eyes closed, over the steam, breathing the steam for no more than 10 minutes at a time.
4. For babies and children younger than 6 years, make a larger tent with a blanket or sheet and sit with them around the bowl.

CONGESTION-RELIEVING HUMIDIFIER BLEND

MAKES ½ OUNCE ❧ AROMATIC

1 teaspoon fir needle essential oil
¾ teaspoon lemon essential oil

¾ teaspoon rosalina essential oil
½ teaspoon cypress essential oil

TO MAKE THE BLEND

Add all the essential oils to an empty essential oil bottle (or any dark glass bottle with a dropper), and gently swirl the bottle to combine.

TO DIFFUSE THE BLEND

Add the recommended drops to the humidifier water and diffuse throughout the room in 30-minute increments (30 minutes on/30 minutes off).

0–6 mo.	6–24 mo.	2–6 yr.	6+ yr.
2 drops	4 drops	6 drops	8 drops

DECONGESTING AROMATHERAPY INHALER

MAKES 1 TREATMENT ❧ AROMATIC

	3–6 mo.	6–24 mo.	2–6 yr.	6+ yr.
Fir needle essential oil	5 drops	5 drops	10 drops	10 drops
Frankincense essential oil	no drops	2 drops	5 drops	5 drops
Rosalina essential oil	5 drops	3 drops	5 drops	5 drops

1. Combine all the essential oils in a small glass bowl.
2. Using tweezers, add the wick (the cotton pad) of an aromatherapy personal inhaler to the bowl and roll it around until it's soaked up all of the essential oils mixture.

3. Use the tweezers to transfer the wick to the inhaler tube. Close the tube and label the inhaler.

4. Let your child take a whiff of the inhaler whenever congestion affects them.

Constipation

Young children often get constipation for many reasons—from dietary issues to stress during potty training. Drinking plenty of water and eating lots of fresh fruits and vegetables will keep things moving along regularly. Essential oils can help relieve some of the pain and gas that goes along with constipation. Some essential oils that help with constipation are dill weed, chamomile, spearmint, ginger, sweet orange, lemon, frankincense, petitgrain, and coriander.

ABDOMINAL MASSAGE OIL #1
MAKES 4 OUNCES ⇒ TOPICAL

	3–6 mo.	6–24 mo.	2–6 yr.	6+ yr.
Unrefined coconut oil	½ cup	½ cup	½ cup	½ cup
Dill weed essential oil	no drops	3 drops	5 drops	7 drops
Roman chamomile essential oil	2 drops	5 drops	10 drops	15 drops
Sweet orange essential oil	2 drops	10 drops	15 drops	20 drops

1. In a small pan over low heat, melt the coconut oil.

2. Once melted, remove from heat, add the dill weed, Roman chamomile, and sweet orange essential oils, and stir to combine.

3. Pour into a Mason jar, and put into the freezer for 20 minutes to harden.

4. Apply a small amount to your child's abdomen and massage in. Store any unused oil in a cool, dark location.

ABDOMINAL MASSAGE OIL #2

MAKES 4 OUNCES ❧ TOPICAL ❧ PHOTOSENSITIZING

	3–6 mo.	6–24 mo.	2–6 yr.	6+ yr.
Unrefined coconut oil	½ cup	½ cup	½ cup	½ cup
Coriander essential oil	no drops	5 drops	10 drops	15 drops
Lemon essential oil	no drops	10 drops	15 drops	20 drops
Spearmint essential oil	no drops	5 drops	10 drops	15 drops

1. In a small pan over low heat, melt the coconut oil.
2. Once melted, remove from heat, add the coriander, lemon, and spearmint essential oils, and stir to combine.
3. Pour into a Mason jar, and put into the freezer for 20 minutes to harden.
4. Apply a small amount to your child's abdomen and massage in. Store any unused oil in a cool, dark location.

SAFETY TIP Lemon essential oil is photosensitizing, so if you are using this remedy, be sure your child's abdomen is covered up before going out into the sun.

Cough

There are two types of coughs—dry and wet. Dry coughs are characterized by intense bouts of spastic coughing and/or a tickling of the throat, and require calming and soothing. Wet coughs are characterized by the constant production of mucus and phlegm, which need to be expelled. A chest rub-diffuser combo works to ease breathing so kids can get rest. (For children younger than 3 months, diffusion is recommended.) Anti-inflammatory and expectorant essential oils including lavender, rosalina, fir needle, tea tree, palmarosa, cypress, pine, marjoram, chamomile, spearmint, frankincense, petitgrain, spruce, sandalwood, and ginger soothe irritation, calm coughing, and open up the airways.

COUGH DIFFUSER BLEND
MAKES ½ OUNCE ➤ AROMATIC

1 teaspoon fir needle essential oil
1 teaspoon rosalina essential oil

½ teaspoon lavender essential oil
½ teaspoon petitgrain essential oil

TO MAKE THE BLEND

Add all the essential oils to an empty essential oil bottle (or any dark glass bottle with a dropper), and gently swirl the bottle to combine.

TO DIFFUSE THE BLEND

Add the recommended drops to a diffuser and diffuse throughout the room in 30-minute increments (30 minutes on/30 minutes off).

0–6 mo.	6–24 mo.	2–6 yr.	6+ yr.
2 drops	4 drops	6 drops	8 drops

DRY COUGH CHEST RUB
MAKES 4 OUNCES ➤ TOPICAL

	3–6 mo.	6–24 mo.	2–6 yr.	6+ yr.
Unrefined coconut oil	½ cup	½ cup	½ cup	½ cup
Fir needle essential oil	2 drops	10 drops	16 drops	20 drops
Lavender essential oil	2 drops	4 drops	10 drops	15 drops
Sweet marjoram essential oil	no drops	4 drops	10 drops	15 drops

1. In a small pan over low heat, melt the coconut oil.
2. Once melted, remove from heat, and add the fir needle, lavender, and sweet marjoram essential oils. ➤

3. Pour into a 4-ounce Mason jar, and put into the freezer for 20 minutes to harden.
4. Rub onto your baby's chest, back, and the bottoms of their feet. Cover the feet with socks. Store the rub in a cool, dark location.

SAFETY TIP Do not apply chest rub to the child's face or under their nose.

EXPECTORANT CHEST RUB
MAKES 4 OUNCES ❧ TOPICAL

	3–6 mo.	6–24 mo.	2–6 yr.	6+ yr.
Unrefined coconut oil	½ cup	½ cup	½ cup	½ cup
Lavender essential oil	2 drops	4 drops	10 drops	15 drops
Rosalina essential oil	2 drops	10 drops	15 drops	20 drops
Tea tree essential oil	no drops	4 drops	10 drops	15 drops

1. In a small pan over low heat, melt the coconut oil.
2. Once melted, remove from heat, and add the lavender, rosalina, and tea tree essential oils.
3. Pour into a 4-ounce Mason jar, and put into the freezer for 20 minutes to harden.
4. Rub onto your baby's chest, back, and the bottoms of their feet. Cover the feet with socks. Store the rub in a cool, dark location.

HELPFUL HINT For babies over 1 year, 1 teaspoon of raw unfiltered honey is a fantastic expectorant and throat soother. (Never feed honey to babies under 1 year old.)

Cradle Cap

Caused by overactive sebaceous glands, cradle cap is a common condition in newborns producing crusty or oily scaly patches on a baby's scalp, eyebrows, and behind the ears. Cradle cap doesn't irritate baby and can easily be removed with natural remedies. Don't use essential oils topically on babies under 3 months of age. Instead hydrosols are the way to go. Applying coconut oil to all the affected areas and softly brushing away the scales is also effective.

CRADLE CAP HEAD WASH
MAKES 4 OUNCES ❧ SAFE FOR ALL AGES

¼ cup plus 2 tablespoons lavender hydrosol

1 tablespoon aloe vera gel

1 tablespoon vegetable glycerin

1. Add all the ingredients to a 4-ounce spray bottle. Gently swirl the bottle to combine.
2. To use, spray your baby's scalp and brush with a gentle baby brush. Gently pat dry and follow with coconut oil or Lavender-Coconut Cradle Cap Conditioner (below).

LAVENDER-COCONUT CRADLE CAP CONDITIONER
MAKES 4 OUNCES ❧ SAFE FOR ALL AGES

¼ cup unrefined coconut oil

2 tablespoons lavender buds

2 tablespoons unrefined shea butter

1 tablespoon beeswax pastilles

1 tablespoon hemp seed oil

1. In a small pan over low heat, combine the coconut oil and lavender buds and steep for 1 to 3 hours. Strain.
2. In the same small pan over low heat, add the lavender-coconut oil, shea butter, beeswax, and hemp seed oil. Once melted, remove from heat.
3. Pour into a Mason jar, and put into the freezer for 20 minutes to harden.
4. Apply to your baby's scalp at least once a day, especially after washing your baby's hair, until cradle cap is gone. Store any unused conditioner in a cool, dark location when not in use.

Croup

Croup, a common respiratory condition in young children usually caused by a virus that inflames the airways, is characterized by a barking cough. Most common in babies and young children, croup can be treated using antiviral essential oils that help to open up the airways and reduce inflammation, including lavender, chamomile, marjoram, tea tree, ginger, black pepper, rosalina, fir needle, cypress, lemon, frankincense, spruce, cedarwood, palmarosa, pine, and sandalwood. If your child is having trouble catching their breath or their breathing is obstructed, seek medical attention immediately.

CROUP DIFFUSER BLEND

MAKES ½ OUNCE ➤ AROMATIC ➤ PHOTOSENSITZING

1 teaspoon marjoram essential oil

¾ teaspoon fir needle essential oil

¾ teaspoon lemon essential oil

¾ teaspoon tea tree essential oil

TO MAKE THE BLEND

Add all the essential oils to an empty essential oil bottle (or any dark glass bottle with a dropper), and gently swirl the bottle to combine.

TO DIFFUSE THE BLEND

Add the recommended drops to a diffuser and diffuse throughout the room in 30-minute increments (30 minutes on/30 minutes off).

0–6 mo.	6–24 mo.	2–6 yr.	6+ yr.
2 drops	4 drops	6 drops	8 drops

HELPFUL HINT This essential oil blend can be used in a chest rub diluted in coconut oil or even added to a humidifier in your bedroom. This blend contains photosensitizing lemon essential oil, so don't forget to dilute before using topically and use caution in the sun.

KICK THE CROUP CHEST RUB
MAKES ABOUT 4 OUNCES ❧ TOPICAL ❧ AROMATIC

	3–6 mo.	6–24 mo.	2–6 yr.	6+ yr.
Unrefined coconut oil	½ cup	½ cup	½ cup	½ cup
Cypress essential oil	no drops	5 drops	10 drops	15 drops
Roman chamomile essential oil	2 drops	5 drops	10 drops	15 drops
Rosalina essential oil	2 drops	10 drops	15 drops	20 drops

1. In a small pan over low heat, melt the coconut oil.
2. Once melted, remove from heat, add the cypress, Roman chamomile, and rosalina essential oils, and stir to combine.
3. Pour into a Mason jar, and put into the freezer for 20 minutes to harden.
4. Apply to your baby's chest, back, neck, and the bottoms of their feet. Cover the feet with socks. Store any unused rub in a cool, dark location.

Cuts and Scrapes

Boo-boos and owies are a normal part of childhood, but infected wounds and scars needn't be. Most essential oils have some sort of antibacterial or antiseptic properties, making them perfect for an antiseptic owie cream or a cleansing owie wash. Antibacterial and skin-healing essential oils such as lavender, chamomile, tea tree, geranium, neroli, frankincense, palmarosa, rose, helichrysum, sandalwood, blue tansy, cedarwood, fir needle, cypress, and sweet orange are all effective at soothing the pain of owies while healing them up and preventing infection.

ANTIBACTERIAL CLEANSING OWIE SPRAY

MAKES ABOUT 4 OUNCES ⇒ TOPICAL

	3–6 mo.	6–24 mo.	2–6 yr.	6+ yr.
Witch hazel	2 tbsp.	2 tbsp.	2 tbsp.	2 tbsp.
Aloe vera	1 tbsp.	1 tbsp.	1 tbsp.	1 tbsp.
Vegetable glycerin	1 tsp.	1 tsp.	1 tsp.	1 tsp.
German chamomile essential oil	no drops	2 drops	4 drops	6 drops
Lavender essential oil	4 drops	4 drops	6 drops	10 drops
Tea tree essential oil	no drops	4 drops	6 drops	10 drops
Distilled water	to fill	to fill	to fill	to fill

1. In a 4-ounce spray bottle, combine the witch hazel, aloe vera gel, and vegetable glycerin with the German chamomile, lavender, and tea tree essential oils. Gently swirl to mix.

2. Add enough distilled water to fill the bottle.

3. To use, spray onto boo-boos and owies. Gently pat dry with a clean cloth or towel. Follow with Healing Antiseptic Boo-Boo Balm (page 161). Store any unused spray in a cool, dark location.

SUBSTITUTION TIP For extra skin- and scar-healing benefits, substitute calendula or chamomile hydrosol for the water in this recipe. Both chamomile and calendula are well known for their abilities to soothe inflammation, boost tissue regeneration, and heal wounds.

HEALING ANTISEPTIC BOO-BOO BALM

MAKES ABOUT 4 OUNCES ⇝ TOPICAL ⇝ PHOTOSENSITIZING

	3–6 mo.	6–24 mo.	2–6 yr.	6+ yr.
Unrefined coconut oil	¼ cup	¼ cup	¼ cup	¼ cup
Beeswax pastilles	2 tbsp.	2 tbsp.	2 tbsp.	2 tbsp.
Unrefined shea butter	2 tbsp.	2 tbsp.	2 tbsp.	2 tbsp.
Lavender essential oil	4 drops	8 drops	15 drops	20 drops
Lemon essential oil	no drops	4 drops	10 drops	15 drops
Tea tree essential oil	no drops	8 drops	15 drops	20 drops

1. In a small pan over low heat, melt the coconut oil, beeswax, and shea butter.
2. Once melted, remove from heat, and add the lavender, lemon, and tea tree essential oils.
3. Pour into a Mason jar, and put into the freezer for 20 minutes to harden.
4. Apply the salve to clean boo-boos whenever needed. Store any unused balm in a cool, dark location.

AWESOME ADDITION Calendula and plantain are herbs well known for their anti-inflammatory and skin-healing properties. Steep 2 tablespoons of herbs in the coconut oil over low heat for 2 hours. Strain before continuing with the recipe.

SAFETY TIP Lemon essential oil is photosensitizing, so be sure and keep any boo-boos and owies treated with this remedy out of the sun. In general, keeping small scrapes out of the sun also lessens scarring.

Dandruff

Children can get dandruff—flakes of dead skin appearing on the scalp, hair, and shoulders—for many different reasons, including dry skin, shampooing too much, chemical sensitivities, eczema, psoriasis, or even a fungal infection. Antifungal and skin-healing essential oils such as lavender, tea tree, palmarosa, sweet orange, lemon, cedarwood, fir needle, rosalina, chamomile, patchouli, cinnamon leaf, clary sage, bergamot, grapefruit, tangerine, sandalwood, geranium, petitgrain, and coriander can help to eliminate dandruff and soothe the scalp.

DANDRUFF SHAMPOO ADD-IN
MAKES ½ OUNCE ❧ TOPICAL

1 teaspoon sweet orange essential oil

1 teaspoon palmarosa essential oil

1 teaspoon tea tree essential oil

1. Add all the essential oils to an empty essential oil bottle (or any dark glass bottle with a dropper), and gently swirl the bottle to combine. Don't forget to label your creation.

2. Add the recommended drops to 8 ounces of shampoo.

3–6 mo.	6–24 mo.	2–6 yr.	6+ yr.
no drops (see Substitution Tip)	10 drops	15 drops	20 drops

SUBSTITUTION TIP For babies 3 to 6 months of age, use 5 drops of lavender essential oil in 8 ounces of shampoo.

DANDRUFF CONDITIONING SPRAY

MAKES ABOUT 8 OUNCES ⇝ TOPICAL

	3–6 mo.	6–24 mo.	2–6 yr.	6+ yr.
Distilled water	½ cup	½ cup	½ cup	½ cup
Marshmallow root	¼ cup	¼ cup	¼ cup	¼ cup
Raw unfiltered apple cider vinegar	1 tbsp.	1 tbsp.	1 tbsp.	1 tbsp.
Aloe vera gel	3 tbsp.	3 tbsp.	3 tbsp.	3 tbsp.
Lavender essential oil	2 drops	5 drops	10 drops	15 drops
Lemon essential oil	no drops	3 drops	5 drops	7 drops
Filtered water	to fill	to fill	to fill	to fill

1. Pour the distilled water in a small bowl and add the marshmallow root. Steep overnight at room temperature. Strain through a fine mesh strainer.
2. In an 8-ounce spray bottle, combine the marshmallow root tea, apple cider vinegar, aloe vera gel, and the lavender and lemon essential oils. Gently swirl to combine.
3. Add enough filtered water to fill the bottle.
4. Shake well before use. Spray onto the scalp and hair, and comb through. Store any unused spray in the refrigerator.

SUBSTITUTION TIP Lavender is naturally antifungal and great at healing most skin conditions. Lavender hydrosol would make a fantastic substitute for the filtered water in this recipe.

Diaper Rash

Diaper rash can be caused by allergic reactions to chemicals in the diapers, wipes, or creams being applied to a baby's bottom. It can also be caused by a fungal infection, eczema, or psoriasis. Antibacterial, antifungal, and skin-healing essential oils such as lavender, chamomile, tea tree, rosalina, palmarosa, lemon, sweet orange, frankincense, geranium, neroli, petitgrain, blue tansy can help to soothe the pain and heal up diaper rash.

BABY BUTT BALM
MAKES ABOUT 4 OUNCES ❧ TOPICAL

	3–6 mo.	6–24 mo.	2–6 yr.	6+ yr.
Unrefined coconut oil	½ cup	½ cup	½ cup	½ cup
Beeswax pastilles	2 tbsp.	2 tbsp.	2 tbsp.	2 tbsp.
Unrefined shea butter	2 tbsp.	2 tbsp.	2 tbsp.	2 tbsp.
German chamomile essential oil	2 drops	10 drops	15 drops	20 drops
Lavender essential oil	2 drops	10 drops	15 drops	20 drops

1. In a small pan over low heat, melt the coconut oil, beeswax, and shea butter.
2. Once melted, remove the pan from the heat. Add the German chamomile and lavender essential oils.
3. Pour into a Mason jar, and put into the freezer for 20 minutes to harden.
4. Apply the salve to itchy skin and rashes whenever needed. Store any unused balm in a cool, dark location.

SAFETY TIP This salve can be made without essential oils for babies under 3 months of age. Try steeping the coconut oil with 2 tablespoons lavender buds or calendula flowers before using in this recipe.

ANTIBACTERIAL BABY BUM WASH SPRAY

MAKES ABOUT 4 OUNCES ⤳ TOPICAL

	3–6 mo.	6–24 mo.	2–6 yr.	6+ yr.
Witch hazel	2 tbsp.	2 tbsp.	2 tbsp.	2 tbsp.
Aloe vera gel	1 tbsp.	1 tbsp.	1 tbsp.	1 tbsp.
Vegetable glycerin	1 tsp.	1 tsp.	1 tsp.	1 tsp.
Blue tansy essential oil	1 drop	2 drops	3 drops	4 drops
Lavender essential oil	2 drops	5 drops	7 drops	10 drops
Filtered water	to fill	to fill	to fill	to fill

1. Add the witch hazel, aloe vera gel, vegetable glycerin, and the blue tansy and lavender essential oils to a 4-ounce spray bottle. Gently swirl the bottle to combine.

2. Add enough filtered water to fill the bottle.

3. To use, spray onto baby's bottom and gently pat dry with a clean cloth or towel. Follow with Baby Butt Balm (page 164). Store any unused spray in a cool, dark location.

SUBSTITUTION TIP For extra skin-healing benefits, substitute calendula or chamomile hydrosol for the water in this recipe. Both chamomile and calendula are well known for their abilities to soothe inflammation, boost tissue regeneration, and heal wounds.

SOOTHING HOMEMADE BABY WIPES

MAKES 24 WIPES ⇒ TOPICAL

	3–6 mo.	6–24 mo.	2–6 yr.	6+ yr.
Unrefined coconut oil	1 tbsp.	1 tbsp.	1 tbsp.	1 tbsp.
Lavender essential oil	5 drops	5 drops	10 drops	10 drops
Tea tree essential oil	5 drops	5 drops	10 drops	10 drops
Filtered water	½ cup	½ cup	½ cup	½ cup
Aloe vera gel	1 tbsp.	1 tbsp.	1 tbsp.	1 tbsp.

1. In a small pan over low heat, melt the coconut oil. Remove from heat, add the lavender and tea tree essential oils, and stir to combine.

2. Cut 12 paper towels in half and stack them in a glass container that has a lid. Whisk the filtered water and aloe vera gel into the coconut oil mixture, then pour over the stack of paper towels. The paper towels should soak up all the liquid.

3. Cover the wipes with the lid, and store in the refrigerator when not using for up to 1 month.

SAFETY TIP For babies under 3 months of age, omit the essential oils from this recipe and substitute lavender or chamomile hydrosol for the water.

Diarrhea

Watery loose stool, or diarrhea, has a number of causes including a cold, the flu, ear infections, bacterial and viral stomach infections, stress, or even allergic reactions to food or medicine. It is very important to keep your child hydrated when they have diarrhea. Digestive and antiviral essential oils such as lavender, chamomile, spearmint, ginger, lemon, sweet orange, petitgrain, and dill weed can help to calm and soothe upset tummies and relieve stress.

STRESS-RELIEVING TUMMY TAMER RUB
MAKES ABOUT 1 OUNCE ⇒ TOPICAL

	3–6 mo.	6–24 mo.	2–6 yr.	6+ yr.
Unrefined coconut oil	2 tbsp.	2 tbsp.	2 tbsp.	2 tbsp.
Lavender essential oil	no drops	1 drop	3 drops	5 drops
Roman chamomile essential oil	1 drop	2 drops	4 drops	6 drops
Tangerine essential oil	no drops	1 drop	2 drops	2 drops

1. In a small pan over low heat, melt the coconut oil.
2. Once melted, remove from heat. Add the lavender, Roman chamomile, and tangerine essential oils, and stir to combine.
3. Pour into a Mason jar, and put into the freezer for 20 minutes to harden.
4. Apply a small amount to your child's abdomen and gently massage in. Store any unused rub in a cool, dark location.

PEPPERMINT ELECTROLYTE LEMONADE
MAKES ABOUT 28 OUNCES ⇒ SAFE FOR ALL AGES

3 cups filtered water
1 cup peppermint hydrosol
½ cup freshly squeezed lemon juice

Maple syrup to taste
¼ teaspoon sea salt

1. In a pitcher, mix all the ingredients together until the salt and syrup are completely dissolved. ➔

2. Have your kids drink this beverage to rehydrate during illness. Store any leftovers in the refrigerator.

AWESOME ADDITION Activated charcoal is widely used in hospitals across the United States to treat food, drug, and chemical poisoning. If taken immediately after the poisonous substance is ingested, the charcoal can absorb and neutralize it. If food poisoning is suspected, stir ½ teaspoon activated charcoal into the lemonade. While it will turn the beverage black, it will not change the taste. *However, if you suspect your child has ingested dangerous chemicals, such as household cleaners, poisonous plants, or medicine, call 911.*

ANTIVIRAL TUMMY TAMER RUB
MAKES ABOUT 1 OUNCE ➤ TOPICAL

	3–6 mo.	6–24 mo.	2–6 yr.	6+ yr.
Unrefined coconut oil	2 tbsp.	2 tbsp.	2 tbsp.	2 tbsp.
Ginger essential oil	no drops	no drops	3 drops	6 drops
Lavender essential oil	1 drop	3 drops	3 drops	6 drops
Petitgrain essential oil	no drops	2 drops	3 drops	6 drops

1. In a small pan over low heat, melt the coconut oil.
2. Once melted, remove from heat. Add the ginger, lavender, and petitgrain essential oils, and stir to combine.
3. Pour into a Mason jar, and put into the freezer for 20 minutes to harden.
4. Apply a small amount to your child's abdomen and gently massage in. Store any unused tub in a cool, dark location.

Dry Skin

Dry skin is caused by anything from weather, sunburns, and overuse of soap, to eczema, psoriasis, and fungal issues. Applying a good body butter or other type of moisturizer immediately after a bath or shower helps put moisture back into the skin. Pat skin dry instead of wiping after bathing, and follow with your favorite moisturizer. Carrier oils like hemp seed oil or coconut oil and butters including shea and mango are healing, moisturizing, and soften skin. Skin-healing essential oils include lavender, chamomile, sweet orange, neroli, geranium, rosalina, frankincense, patchouli, petitgrain, palmarosa, helichrysum, sandalwood, coriander, bergamot, grapefruit, lemon, cedarwood, blue tansy, carrot seed, and rose.

ULTRA MOISTURIZING BODY BUTTER
MAKES ABOUT 4 OUNCES ❧ TOPICAL

	3–6 mo.	6–24 mo.	2–6 yr.	6+ yr.
Unrefined shea butter	¼ cup	¼ cup	¼ cup	¼ cup
Unrefined coconut oil	2 tbsp.	2 tbsp.	2 tbsp.	2 tbsp.
Hemp seed oil	2 tbsp.	2 tbsp.	2 tbsp.	2 tbsp.
Lavender essential oil	2 drops	10 drops	15 drops	20 drops
Sweet orange essential oil	2 drops	10 drops	15 drops	20 drops

1. In a double boiler or in a metal mixing bowl over a pan of hot water, melt the shea butter and coconut oil.
2. Once melted, remove from heat. Add the hemp seed oil and the lavender and sweet orange essential oils.

3. For simple, hard body butter, pour the melted mixture into a tin or jar, and put into the freezer for 20 minutes, to harden. For whipped body butter, cool the bowl over an ice bath until the butter is mostly hardened with a little pool of liquid on top, and then whip with a hand mixer until light and fluffy. It will continue to thicken overnight as it cools completely. Store unused butter in a cool, dark location.

MOISTURIZING BODY OIL
MAKES ABOUT 4 OUNCES → TOPICAL

	3–6 mo.	6–24 mo.	2–6 yr.	6+ yr.
Unrefined coconut oil	3 tbsp.	3 tbsp.	3 tbsp.	3 tbsp.
Hemp seed oil	¼ cup	¼ cup	¼ cup	¼ cup
Argan oil	1 tbsp.	1 tbsp.	1 tbsp.	1 tbsp.
Neroli essential oil	2 drops	5 drops	10 drops	15 drops
Sweet orange essential oil	2 drops	5 drops	10 drops	15 drops

1. In a small pan over low heat, melt the coconut oil.
2. Once melted, remove from heat, add the hemp seed oil, argan oil, and the neroli and sweet orange essential oils, and stir to combine.
3. Pour into a Mason jar, and store any unused oil in a cool, dark location.

Earaches and Ear Infection

It is a common misconception that antibiotics should be given at the first sign of an ear infection. Most ear infections are viral, and not bacterial, making the antibiotic prescription worthless. Even the Centers for Disease Control has concluded that "ear infections will often get better on their own without antibiotic treatment." And other studies have shown that using antibiotics unnecessarily can be harmful. Essential oils such as lavender, chamomile, rosalina, palmarosa, tea tree, marjoram, and frankincense can help reduce inflammation and soothe pain caused by an ear infection, while aiding your body in fighting the virus.

SOOTHING GARLIC EAR OIL
MAKES 4 OUNCES ⁓ TOPICAL

	3–6 mo.	6–24 mo.	2–6 yr.	6+ yr.
Fresh garlic, minced	3 cloves	3 cloves	3 cloves	3 cloves
Extra-virgin olive oil	½ cup	½ cup	½ cup	½ cup
Lavender essential oil	2 drop	3 drops	6 drops	9 drops
Palmarosa essential oil	no drops	1 drop	3 drops	3 drops
Rosalina essential oil	no drops	1 drop	3 drops	3 drops

1. In a small pan over low heat, combine the olive oil and minced garlic. Steep the garlic in the oil over low heat for 1 to 3 hours.
2. Remove the pan from the heat. Using a fine mesh sieve or cheesecloth, strain the oil into a glass bowl taking great care not to leave any pieces of garlic in the strained oil.
3. Add the lavender, palmarosa, and rosalina essential oils and swirl gently to combine. Store in a dark glass bottle with a dropper. ➔

4. To use, warm the bottle by either placing it in a bowl of warm water for 3 to 5 minutes, rubbing the bottle between your hands until warm, or first running the outside of the dropper under warm water and then quickly drying before sucking up oil. Be sure to test the oil on your forearm, as you would warmed baby bath or milk. Drop 2 to 3 drops of warm oil into each ear every 4 hours as needed. Always treat both ears because ear infections can move from ear to ear.

SAFETY TIP This remedy is not effective for "swimmer's ear" and other infections caused by water entering the ear; in fact, the remedy can make those types of infections worse. If dealing with a perforated eardrum, do not use this remedy; nothing should be poured into the ear. To be able to know what is going on inside of your child's ear, pick up a Dr. Mom Otoscope (DrMomOtoscope.com) for your medicine chest.

EAR AND NECK MASSAGE OIL
MAKES 2 OUNCES ⚬ TOPICAL

	3–6 mo.	6–24 mo.	2–6 yr.	6+ yr.
Unrefined coconut oil	¼ cup	¼ cup	¼ cup	¼ cup
German chamomile essential oil	1 drop	1 drop	2 drops	4 drops
Lavender essential oil	2 drops	4 drops	6 drops	8 drops
Rosalina essential oil	1 drop	2 drops	4 drops	6 drops

1. In a small pan over low heat, melt the coconut oil.
2. Once melted, remove from heat, add the German chamomile, lavender, and rosalina essential oils, and stir to combine.
3. Pour into a Mason jar, and put into the freezer for 20 minutes to harden.
4. Apply a small amount around the ears and neck, massaging in. Store any unused oil in a cool, dark location.

Eczema and Psoriasis

Food allergies or sensitivities are partially responsible for most cases of eczema, though it can present with medications and body care product sensitivities as well. For many, eating lots of foods with omega-3 fatty acids, fermented foods, and foods high in good fats (avocados, coconuts) can be the key to completely healing eczema. Both eczema and psoriasis respond well to essential oils. Anti-inflammatory and skin-healing essential oils including lavender, neroli, palmarosa, chamomile, blue tansy, cedarwood, geranium, coriander, frankincense, tea tree, rosalina, sandalwood, patchouli, and helichrysum can help to reduce inflammation, increase cell regeneration, and soothe and heal both eczema and psoriasis breakouts.

SKIN-SOOTHING SALVE
MAKES ABOUT 4 OUNCES ❧ TOPICAL

	3–6 mo.	6–24 mo.	2–6 yr.	6+ yr.
Unrefined coconut oil	¼ cup	¼ cup	¼ cup	¼ cup
Beeswax pastilles	2 tbsp.	2 tbsp.	2 tbsp.	2 tbsp.
Unrefined shea butter	2 tbsp.	2 tbsp.	2 tbsp.	2 tbsp.
Atlas cedarwood essential oil	no drops	5 drops	10 drops	15 drops
Lavender essential oil	4 drops	10 drops	15 drops	20 drops
Palmarosa essential oil	no drops	5 drops	10 drops	15 drops

1. In a small pan over low heat, melt the coconut oil, beeswax, and shea butter.
2. Once melted, remove from heat, and add the Atlas cedarwood, lavender, and palmarosa essential oils.
3. Pour into a Mason jar, and put into the freezer for 20 minutes to harden.

4. Apply the salve whenever a breakout occurs. Store any unused salve in a cool, dark location.

AWESOME ADDITION Calendula is well known for its skin-healing, anti-inflammatory properties and would make a great addition to this salve. Steep 2 tablespoons of herb in the coconut oil over low heat for 2 hours. Strain and continue with the recipe.

SOOTHING SKIN SOAPLESS HERBAL BODY WASH
MAKES ABOUT 8 OUNCES ≫ SAFE FOR ALL AGES ≫ TOPICAL

¾ cup lavender or chamomile hydrosol

3 to 4 soap nuts

1 tablespoon marshmallow root

2 tablespoons aloe vera gel

2 tablespoons witch hazel

1. In a small pan over medium heat, heat the hydrosol, soap nuts, and marshmallow root.
2. Bring the mixture to a boil, then decrease the heat and simmer for 20 minutes.
3. Remove from heat and steep while the mixture cools to room temperature.
4. Once cool, strain the herbs using a fine mesh sieve or cheesecloth.
5. Combine the herbal tea infusion with the aloe vera gel and witch hazel. Store in the refrigerator up to a week.

HELPFUL TIP A member of the lychee family, soap nuts are berries that grow on the soapberry tree (genus *Sapindus*) and contain saponins, a natural surfactant. Soapberry trees can be found all over the world, including Asia and the Americas. Used for centuries to clean clothing, hair, and bodies, soap nuts are a great eco-friendly option over many of the toxic chemical-laden detergents out there. Soap nuts, unlike commercial soaps with artificial foaming agents, do not bubble or foam up when cleaning with them. You can purchase soap nuts on the Internet, but Mountain Rose Herbs (MountainRoseHerbs.com) is my trusted source.

Fevers

It's a common misconception that fevers should be immediately reduced—they have a purpose. Fevers are a natural reaction to fighting infections. Infants younger than 4 months old with a rectal temperature of 100.4°F or above should have their doctor contacted, or go to the ER as the high fever could be a sign of a potentially life-threatening infection. If your child's fever is above 104°F, go to the emergency room, as high fevers can cause seizures in young children. Cooling antiviral and immune-supporting essential oils such as lavender, chamomile, spearmint, rosalina, fir needle, cypress, lemon, sweet orange, neroli, petitgrain, palmarosa, tea tree, grapefruit, coriander, and marjoram can help make your child comfortable while the fever runs its course and ease the symptoms of a fever.

COOLING FEVER COMPRESS
MAKES 1 TREATMENT ⇥ TOPICAL

	3–6 mo.	6–24 mo.	2–6 yr.	6+ yr.
Peppermint tea	1 bag or 1 tbsp.	1 bag or 1 tbsp.	1 bag or 1 tbsp.	1 bag or 1 tbsp.
Lavender essential oil	2 drops	2 drops	2 drops	2 drops
Lemon essential oil	no drops	1 drop	1 drop	2 drops
Spearmint essential oil	no drops	no drops	2 drops	2 drops
Aloe vera gel	1 tbsp.	1 tbsp.	1 tbsp.	1 tbsp.
Raw apple cider vinegar	¼ cup	¼ cup	¼ cup	¼ cup
Water	2 cups	2 cups	2 cups	2 cups

1. Combine 2 cups boiling water with the peppermint tea bag. Cover and steep 15 to 20 minutes. ➔

2. Stir in 1 to 2 cups ice cubes, until the ice is melted and the water temperature is cool, but not ice cold.
3. In a separate small bowl, combine the essential oils and aloe vera gel, and stir to combine.
4. Mix the aloe mixture and apple cider vinegar into the cool peppermint tea and stir to combine.
5. To use, dip a washcloth into the mixture, squeeze out until damp. Apply to the forehead and feet to help draw heat from the body.

FEVER REDUCER BATH
MAKES 1 TREATMENT ❧ TOPICAL

	3–6 mo.	6–24 mo.	2–6 yr.	6+ yr.
Coriander essential oil	no drops	1 drop	2 drops	2 drops
Lavender essential oil	1 drop	1 drop	2 drops	2 drops
Roman chamomile essential oil	1 drop	1 drop	2 drops	2 drops
Aloe vera gel	2 tbsp.	2 tbsp.	2 tbsp.	2 tbsp.
Epsom salt	1 cup	1 cup	1 cup	1 cup
Raw apple cider vinegar	1 cup	1 cup	1 cup	1 cup

1. In a small bowl, stir together the coriander, lavender, and Roman chamomile essential oils with the aloe vera gel.
2. Place the Epsom salt and apple cider vinegar in a medium bowl, and stir in the aloe mixture.
3. Pour the mixture under the running bath water as you fill the tub. Have your child soak in the tub for at least 20 minutes.

Germ Killing and Immune Boosting

When your little one catches a cold, the last thing that you want is for it to spread to the rest of the family. Most essential oils have some sort of antibacterial, antiviral, and/or antiseptic properties, making them perfect for killing germs in the air, on surfaces, and boosting the immune system to fight off any potential infections. Essential oils such as lavender, tea tree, lemon, sweet orange, grapefruit, tangerine, mandarin, marjoram, chamomile, palmarosa, fir needle, cypress, frankincense, geranium, coriander, bergamot, cedarwood, helichrysum, rosalina, neroli, petitgrain, and sandalwood all kill germs and help stimulate the immune system.

CLEANSE THE AIR DIFFUSER BLEND
MAKES ½ OUNCE ❧ AROMATIC

1 teaspoon rosalina essential oil

¾ teaspoon cinnamon leaf essential oil

¾ teaspoon lavender essential oil

½ teaspoon fir needle essential oil

TO MAKE THE BLEND

Add all the essential oils to an empty essential oil bottle (or any dark glass bottle with a dropper), and gently swirl to combine.

TO DIFFUSE THE BLEND

Add the recommended drops to a diffuser and diffuse throughout the room in 30-minute increments (30 minutes on/30 minutes off).

0–6 mo.	6–24 mo.	2–6 yr.	6+ yr.
2 drops	4 drops	6 drops	8 drops

IMMUNE STIMULATING AROMATHERAPY ROLL-ON
MAKES ⅓ OUNCE ❧ TOPICAL ❧ AROMATIC

	3–6 mo.	6–24 mo.	2–6 yr.	6+ yr.
Lavender essential oil	1 drop	1 drop	1 drop	2 drops
Marjoram essential oil	no drops	no drops	1 drop	2 drops
Rosalina essential oil	no drops	1 drop	1 drop	2 drops
Fractionated coconut oil	to fill	to fill	to fill	to fill

1. Add the lavender, marjoram, and rosalina essential oils to a ⅓-ounce glass roll-on bottle.
2. Add enough fractionated coconut oil to fill the bottle. Place the roller ball and cap on, and gently swirl to combine. Don't forget to label your creation.
3. To use, roll onto the back of your child's neck, chest, wrists, and the bottoms of their feet whenever needed.

Growing Pains

Though they are called "growing pains," the pains that children ages 3 to 12 get in their arm and leg muscles aren't actually from growth spurts. While doctors don't yet know the cause, the general consensus is that the pains are most likely caused from depletion of minerals and vitamins during running, playing, jumping, and other energy-exerting activities throughout a child's day. The essential oils lavender, rosalina, chamomile, marjoram, cypress, fir needle, turmeric, helichrysum, juniper berry, lemon, petitgrain, and coriander can help to ease the pain and relax the muscles so that your child can get a better night's sleep.

GROWING PAINS RELIEF BATH

MAKES 1 TREATMENT ❧ TOPICAL

	2–6 yr.	6+ yr.
Lavender essential oil	2 drops	2 drops
Roman chamomile essential oil	2 drops	2 drops
Rosalina essential oil	2 drops	2 drops
Liquid castile soap	1 tbsp.	1 tbsp.
Epsom salt	1 cup	1 cup

1. In a small bowl, stir together the lavender, Roman chamomile, and rosalina essential oils with the liquid soap.
2. Place the Epsom salt in a medium bowl, and stir in the soap mixture.
3. Pour the mixture under the running bath water as you fill the tub.

AWESOME ADDITION Anti-inflammatory herbs such as lavender and chamomile make great additions to this bath. Add ¼ cup of each herb to a cloth tea bag or an old, clean sock, and tie closed before tossing into the bathtub.

GROWING PAINS MASSAGE OIL

MAKES ABOUT 4 OUNCES ❧ TOPICAL

	3–6 mo.	6–24 mo.	2–6 yr.	6+ yr.
Carrier oil	½ cup	½ cup	½ cup	½ cup
Lavender essential oil	no drops	no drops	10 drops	15 drops
Marjoram essential oil	no drops	no drops	10 drops	15 drops
Rosalina essential oil	no drops	no drops	15 drops	20 drops

1. In a medium glass bowl, stir together the carrier oil and lavender, marjoram, and rosalina essential oils.

2. Pour the mixture into a lotion pump bottle (or preferred container) and put into the freezer for 20 minutes to harden.

3. Massage the oil into your child's arms and legs whenever needed. Store any unused oil in a cool, dark location.

AWESOME ADDITION Arnica flowers and St. John's wort are herbs well known for their anti-inflammatory and pain relieving properties. Steep 2 tablespoons arnica flowers and 2 tablespoons St. John's wort in the coconut oil over low heat for 2 hours. Strain and continue with the recipe.

Hand, Foot, and Mouth Disease

Hand, foot, and mouth disease is a viral infection that causes blisters in the mouth, on baby's hands, and on the feet. Very contagious, it can be spread by children touching their blisters then touching furniture, toys, or other objects. Usually lasting around 10 days, the virus can be shortened and blisters healed up using essential oils and hydrosols. These include the essential oils of lavender, tea tree, geranium coriander, chamomile, neroli, rosalina, petitgrain, sweet orange, palmarosa, patchouli, sandalwood, and helichrysum.

PEPPERMINT LAVENDER BLISTER RELIEF MOUTHWASH
MAKES 8 OUNCES ⋊ SAFE FOR ALL AGES

½ cup peppermint hydrosol
¼ cup lavender hydrosol
¼ cup filtered water

1 tablespoon raw unfiltered honey
(for infants under 1 year, substitute
maple syrup or vegetable glycerin)

1. Combine all the ingredients in an 8-ounce jar or container. Shake well to combine, until the honey or maple syrup completely dissolves.

2. For children who can spit, have them gargle with this mouthwash before spitting out. For infants, use a cotton swab and gently apply. Store any unused mouthwash in a cool, dark location.

AWESOME ADDITION Thyme is well known for its antiviral properties, especially against hand, foot, and mouth disease. To use it in this mouthwash, steep 1 tablespoon of thyme in the filtered water for 2 hours before adding to the recipe. Strain before using.

HEALING ANTIVIRAL SALVE
MAKES ABOUT 4 OUNCES ⇾ TOPICAL

	3–6 mo.	6–24 mo.	2–6 yr.	6+ yr.
Unrefined coconut oil	½ cup + 2 tbsp.	½ cup + 2 tbsp.	½ cup + 2 tbsp.	½ cup + 2 tbsp.
Beeswax pastilles	2 tbsp.	2 tbsp.	2 tbsp.	2 tbsp.
Geranium essential oil	no drops	5 drops	10 drops	15 drops
Lavender essential oil	2 drops	5 drops	10 drops	15 drops
Rosalina essential oil	2 drops	10 drops	15 drops	20 drops

1. In a small pan over low heat, melt the coconut oil and beeswax.
2. Once melted, remove from heat, and add the geranium, lavender, and rosalina essential oils.
3. Pour into a Mason jar, and put into the freezer for 20 minutes to harden.
4. Apply the salve to affected areas whenever needed. Store the salve in a cool, dark location.

AWESOME ADDITION Calendula and chamomile are well known for their anti-inflammatory and antiviral properties. Steep 2 tablespoons of each herb in the coconut oil over low heat for 2 hours. Strain and continue with the recipe.

Headaches

Headaches are commonly a symptom of other issues within the body, including lack of sleep, inadequate water or food, low blood sugar, hormones, vitamin deficiency, magnesium deficiency, caffeine detox, sugar detox, and even sensitivity to artificial fragrances. While essential oils can help to soothe a headache, it is best to look at the reason for the headache and treat it accordingly. Essential oils that can be helpful to soothe a headache include lavender, spearmint, ginger, chamomile, petitgrain, rosalina, helichrysum, black pepper, blue tansy, neroli, marjoram, fir needle, cypress, juniper berry, and frankincense.

HEADACHE HEALER DIFFUSER BLEND
MAKES ½ OUNCE ❧ AROMATIC

1 teaspoon lavender essential oil
1 teaspoon rosalina essential oil

½ teaspoon helichrysum essential oil
½ teaspoon Roman chamomile essential oil

TO MAKE THE BLEND

Add all the essential oils to an empty essential oil bottle (or any dark glass bottle with a dropper), and gently swirl the bottle to combine.

TO DIFFUSE THE BLEND

Add the recommended drops to a diffuser and diffuse throughout the room in 30-minute increments (30 minutes on/30 minutes off).

0–6 mo.	6–24 mo.	2–6 yr.	6+ yr.
2 drops	4 drops	6 drops	8 drops

HEADACHE MASSAGE OIL

MAKES 1 OUNCE ⪼ TOPICAL

	3–6 mo.	6–24 mo.	2–6 yr.	6+ yr.
Unrefined coconut oil	½ cup	½ cup	½ cup	½ cup
Lavender essential oil	no drops	5 drops	10 drops	15 drops
Rosalina essential oil	no drops	5 drops	10 drops	15 drops
Spearmint essential oil	no drops	10 drops	15 drops	20 drops

1. In a small pan over low heat, melt the coconut oil.
2. Once melted, remove from heat. Add the lavender, rosalina, and spearmint essential oils, and stir to combine.
3. Pour into a Mason jar, and put into the freezer for 20 minutes to harden.
4. Apply a small amount to the temples, back of neck, shoulders, and forehead. Gently massage in. Store any remaining oil in a cool, dark location.

Head Lice

For many moms, the thought of a child acquiring head lice is their worst parental nightmare. Not only do you need to kill the bugs on everyone's heads in your household, but you must get rid of them throughout your house, too—pillows, stuffed animals, and more could be hosting them. Fortunately, you can skip the toxic pesticides because essential oils are great at killing bugs without harming your children or the environment. You can add them to your normal shampoo, make a detangling spray, and even use them in a carpet powder. Essential oils that get rid of head lice include lavender, tea tree, sweet orange, cedarwood, palmarosa, spearmint, rosalina, geranium, and patchouli.

HEAD LICE SHAMPOO ADD-IN BLEND
MAKES ½ OUNCE

1 teaspoon sweet orange essential oil
1 teaspoon tea tree essential oil

½ teaspoon Atlas cedarwood essential oil
½ teaspoon palmarosa essential oil

1. Add all the essential oils to an empty essential oil bottle (or any dark glass bottle with a dropper), and gently swirl the bottle to combine. Don't forget to label your creation.
2. Add the recommended drops to 8 ounces of shampoo.

3–6 mo.	6–24 mo.	2–6 yr.	6+ yr.
5 drops	10 drops	15 drops	20 drops

HELPFUL HINT This undiluted blend can be used diluted in a carrier oil as a head lice scalp oil, or even used diluted in your favorite conditioner for a deep conditioning lice killer. This blend is strong, so don't forget to dilute before using topically.

HEAD LICE SCALP OIL
MAKES 4 OUNCES ➢ TOPICAL

	3–6 mo.	6–24 mo.	2–6 yr.	6+ yr.
Unrefined coconut oil	½ cup	½ cup	½ cup	½ cup
Head Lice Shampoo Add-In Blend (page 184)	4 drops	15 drops	30 drops	50 drops

1. In a small pan over low heat, melt the coconut oil.
2. Once melted, remove from heat, add the recommended drops of the add-in blend, and stir to combine.

3. Pour into a Mason jar, and put into the freezer for 20 minutes to harden.

4. Apply to your child's scalp and cover with a shower cap or plastic wrap. Leave on the scalp for 2 hours before shampooing out. Follow with a nit comb to remove any eggs and lice. Store any unused oil in a cool, dark location.

LICE VACUUM CARPET POWDER

MAKES 1 CUP ❧ SAFE FOR ALL AGES

½ cup food grade diatomaceous earth
½ cup baking soda

30 drops Head Lice Shampoo Add-In Blend (page 184)

1. In a medium bowl, combine the diatomaceous earth and baking soda.

2. Add the add-in blend, stirring to disperse evenly throughout the powder.

3. To use, sprinkle onto the carpet and let sit overnight before vacuuming up. Repeat as needed.

AWESOME ADDITION There are tons of herbs that do a great job repelling and killing bugs. Try mixing ½ cup of finely ground herbs, such as lavender, peppermint, eucalyptus leaves, lemongrass, and rosemary, into the powder to make it even more effective.

HELPFUL TIP Diatomaceous earth (DE) is a chalk-like powder that is made up of diatoms that have fossilized over thousands of years. While DE is safe to use on humans, it is harmful to insects because of its mechanical makeup. It contains no toxins of any kind. On the microscopic level, it is coarse and porous, making it highly absorbent. It sticks to insects and wicks valuable moisture away from their exoskeletons, fatally dehydrating them. This can take time, anywhere from several hours to several days, depending on the conditions and the kind of bug. The great thing about this nontoxic powder is that you can sprinkle it in your garden, around your plants, or even on that line of ants in your kitchen. Just be sure you get food grade DE and not pool grade DE! The pool grade DE can cause respiratory issues. You can purchase my favorite brand at www.DiatomaceousEarth.com.

Heat Rash and Heat Exhaustion

Heat rash and heat exhaustion can occur when your child has been outside in the heat for too long and the body overheats. In the case of heat exhaustion, you should first lay them down, remove most of their clothing, and get them to slowly sip water. Cooling essential oils such as spearmint, chamomile, rosalina, fir needle, blue tansy, cypress, juniper berry, lemon, bergamot, clary sage, and palmarosa can help draw heat from the body when your child is experiencing heat exhaustion. Heat exhaustion can turn into heatstroke. *If heatstroke is suspected, contact your medical practitioner immediately.*

COOLING COMPRESS
MAKES 1 TREATMENT ⊱ TOPICAL

	3–6 mo.	6–24 mo.	2–6 yr.	6+ yr.
German chamomile essential oil	2 drops	2 drops	2 drops	4 drops
Spearmint essential oil	no drops	no drops	2 drops	4 drops
Aloe vera gel	1 tbsp.	1 tbsp.	1 tbsp.	1 tbsp.
Raw apple cider vinegar	¼ cup	¼ cup	¼ cup	¼ cup
Cool water	4 cups	4 cups	4 cups	4 cups

1. In a small glass bowl, stir together the German chamomile and spearmint essential oils with the aloe vera gel. Transfer to a medium bowl.
2. Add the raw apple cider vinegar and cool water, and stir to combine.
3. To use, dip a washcloth into the mixture, squeezing out the excess. Apply to the forehead and feet to help draw heat from the body.

SUBSTITUTION TIP Peppermint tea is well known for its cooling properties and makes a great substitution for the cold water in this recipe. Steep ½ cup of the herb in 4 cups boiling water for 15 to 20 minutes, and let cool completely before substituting in this recipe.

COOL MINT MIST
MAKES ABOUT 8 OUNCES ∾ TOPICAL

	3–6 mo.	6–24 mo.	2–6 yr.	6+ yr.
Peppermint hydrosol	¾ cup + 2 tbsp.	¾ cup + 2 tbsp.	¾ cup + 2 tbsp.	¾ cup + 2 tbsp.
Aloe vera gel	1 tbsp.	1 tbsp.	1 tbsp.	1 tbsp.
Raw unfiltered apple cider vinegar	1 tbsp.	1 tbsp.	1 tbsp.	1 tbsp.
Lemon essential oil	no drops	10 drops	10 drops	10 drops
Spearmint essential oil	no drops	no drops	10 drops	10 drops

1. Combine all the ingredients in an 8-ounce bottle and shake to combine.
2. Shake well before every use. Spray onto the back of your child's neck, chest, and the bottoms of their feet.

HELPFUL HINT I keep this spray in the refrigerator to keep it cooler; it works even better and feels refreshing.

COOL AS A CUCUMBER BATH

MAKES 1 TREATMENT ❧ TOPICAL

	3–6 mo.	6–24 mo.	2–6 yr.	6+ yr.
Cucumber	1	1	1	1
Aloe vera gel	¼ cup	¼ cup	¼ cup	¼ cup
Raw apple cider vinegar	¼ cup	¼ cup	¼ cup	¼ cup
Palmarosa essential oil	no drops	2 drops	5 drops	5 drops
Rosalina essential oil	2 drops	2 drops	2 drops	3 drops
Sea salt	1 cup	1 cup	1 cup	1 cup

1. Blend the cucumber, aloe vera gel, apple cider vinegar, and palmarosa and rosalina essential oils in a blender until completely pureed.
2. Pour the cucumber mixture and sea salt under cool (not cold) running bath water as you fill the tub. Alternately, if you do not want the cucumber floating around, pour the mixture into a fine mesh bag or cloth tea bag while holding it over the closed tub to prevent losing any of the liquid.
3. Have your child soak in the bath until cooled down.

Hives

Raised welts or white lumps on the skin are called *hives*. They are a physical reaction to contact with certain plants, insect bites, or food that causes an allergic reaction on the skin. It is important to get your child's allergies tested so as to avoid inducing the reaction. Essential oils can help reduce the inflammation of the hives as well as relieve some of the itching or pain. Essential oils with anti-inflammatory and antihistamine properties, such as lavender, chamomile, blue tansy, rosalina, tea tree, palmarosa, neroli, helichrysum, and lemon, work well to soothe and heal hives.

ANTI-INFLAMMATORY HIVE RELIEF COMPRESS
MAKES 1 TREATMENT ❯ TOPICAL

	3–6 mo.	6–24 mo.	2–6 yr.	6+ yr.
German chamomile essential oil	1 drop	1 drop	2 drops	3 drops
Lavender essential oil	1 drop	1 drop	2 drops	3 drops
Aloe vera gel	2 tbsp.	2 tbsp.	2 tbsp.	2 tbsp.
Warm water	4 cups	4 cups	4 cups	4 cups
Baking soda	2 tbsp.	2 tbsp.	2 tbsp.	2 tbsp.

1. In a small glass bowl, stir together the essential oils with the aloe vera gel. Transfer to a medium bowl.
2. Add the warm water and baking soda, and stir to combine.
3. To use, dip a washcloth into the mixture, squeezing out the excess. Apply to affected areas.

SUBSTITUTION TIP Chamomile tea is well known for its gentle anti-inflammatory properties and makes a great substitution for the water in this recipe. Steep ½ cup of the herb in 4 cups boiling water for 15 to 20 minutes before substituting.

HIVE RELIEF BEDTIME BODY OIL

MAKES ABOUT 2 OUNCES ❧ TOPICAL

	3–6 mo.	6–24 mo.	2–6 yr.	6+ yr.
Carrier oil	¼ cup	¼ cup	¼ cup	¼ cup
German chamomile essential oil	1 drop	4 drops	5 drops	5 drops
Helichrysum essential oil	no drops	1 drop	5 drops	5 drops
Lavender essential oil	1 drop	5 drops	10 drops	15 drops

Combine all the ingredients in a Mason jar. Apply to affected areas. Store any unused oil in a cool, dark location.

Influenza

Influenza, or flu, is an airborne virus that can last anywhere from 24 hours to 2 weeks depending on the contracted strain. Essential oils can help to kill germs in the air, reduce symptoms to make your child more comfortable, and shorten the life of the virus by boosting the immune system. Antiviral and immune-supporting essential oils including lavender, tea tree, rosalina, frankincense, lemon, sweet orange, bergamot, tangerine, grapefruit, coriander, chamomile, palmarosa, petitgrain, marjoram, cinnamon leaf, fir needle, cypress, juniper berry, and blue tansy can help fight the flu and relieve its symptoms.

FLU FIGHTER DIFFUSER BLEND

MAKES ½ OUNCE ❧ AROMATIC

1 teaspoon lavender essential oil
¾ teaspoon cinnamon leaf essential oil

¾ teaspoon marjoram essential oil
½ teaspoon frankincense essential oil

TO MAKE THE BLEND

Add all the essential oils to an empty essential oil bottle (or any dark glass bottle with a dropper), and gently swirl the bottle to combine.

TO DIFFUSE THE BLEND

Add the recommended drops to a diffuser and diffuse throughout the room in 30-minute increments (30 minutes on/30 minutes off).

0–6 mo.	6–24 mo.	2–6 yr.	6+ yr.
2 drops	4 drops	6 drops	8 drops

FLU FIGHTER CHEST AND BODY RUB
MAKES ABOUT 4 OUNCES ❧ TOPICAL ❧ PHOTOSENSITIZING

	3–6 mo.	6–24 mo.	2–6 yr.	6+ yr.
Unrefined coconut oil	½ cup	½ cup	½ cup	½ cup
Lavender essential oil	4 drops	5 drops	10 drops	15 drops
Lemon essential oil	no drops	5 drops	10 drops	15 drops
Palmarosa essential oil	no drops	10 drops	15 drops	20 drops

1. In a small pan over low heat, melt the coconut oil.
2. Once melted, remove from heat, add the lavender, lemon, and palmarosa essential oils, and stir to combine.
3. Pour into a Mason jar, and put into the freezer for 20 minutes, to harden.
4. Apply a small amount to your child's chest, back of neck, lymph nodes, and the bottoms of their feet. Store any unused rub in a cool, dark location.

Nausea and Vomiting

There are many reasons your child might be nauseated or vomiting, including viral or bacterial infections, food poisoning, or allergies. Hydration, especially with vomiting, is key. Herbal teas are a great source of hydration and valuable nutrients. Lemons are a natural source of electrolytes, vitamin C, and antioxidants. Fresh lemon and ginger tea can keep your child hydrated and soothe their nauseated stomach at the same time. Digestive essential oils such as ginger, spearmint, chamomile, lemon, sweet orange, grapefruit, bergamot, mandarin, tangerine, and dill weed help alleviate nausea and vomiting with just one whiff.

ANTI-NAUSEA INHALER BLEND
MAKES 1 TREATMENT ⇾ AROMATIC

	3–6 mo.	6–24 mo.	2–6 yr.	6+ yr.
Ginger essential oil	no drops	no drops	10 drops	10 drops
Lemon essential oil	no drops	10 drops	5 drops	10 drops
Sweet orange essential oil	15 drops	10 drops	5 drops	10 drops

1. Combine the essential oils in a small glass bowl.
2. Using tweezers, add the wick (the cotton pad) of an aromatherapy personal inhaler to the bowl and roll it around until it's soaked up all of the essential oils mixture.
3. Use the tweezers to transfer the wick to the inhaler tube. Close the tube and label the inhaler.
4. Let your child take a whiff of the inhaler whenever they feel nauseated.

MAKES ½ OUNCE ❧ AROMATIC

1 teaspoon grapefruit essential oil
1 teaspoon spearmint essential oil

1 teaspoon sweet orange
  essential oil

TO MAKE THE BLEND

Add all the essential oils to an empty essential oil bottle (or any dark glass bottle with a dropper), and gently swirl the bottle to combine.

TO DIFFUSE THE BLEND

Add the recommended drops to a diffuser and diffuse throughout the room in 30-minute increments (30 minutes on/30 minutes off).

0–6 mo.	6–24 mo.	2–6 yr.	6+ yr.
2 drops	4 drops	6 drops	8 drops

Pneumonia

Because the symptoms of pneumonia are similar to other chest and sinus infections, it can be difficult to diagnose without a chest x-ray. If you suspect your child has pneumonia, consult with your medical practitioner, as your child may need antibiotics or intensive care. Antiseptic and anti-inflammatory essential oils including lavender, chamomile, fir needle, cypress, rosalina, marjoram, lemon eucalyptus, tea tree, palmarosa, lemon, juniper berry, frankincense, petitgrain, cedarwood, sweet orange, bergamot, coriander, and spearmint can work with medical treatments to ease symptoms, calming the cough and opening up the airways for easier breathing.

BREATHE BETTER DIFFUSER BLEND

MAKES ½ OUNCE ❧ AROMATIC

1 teaspoon fir needle essential oil

1 teaspoon rosalina essential oil

½ teaspoon cypress essential oil

½ teaspoon marjoram essential oil

TO MAKE THE BLEND

Add all the essential oils to an empty essential oil bottle (or any dark glass bottle with a dropper), and gently swirl the bottle to combine.

TO DIFFUSE THE BLEND

Add the recommended drops to a diffuser and diffuse throughout the room in 30-minute increments (30 minutes on/30 minutes off).

0–6 mo.	6–24 mo.	2–6 yr.	6+ yr.
2 drops	4 drops	6 drops	8 drops

PNEUMONIA SHOWER SOOTHERS

MAKES 12 SHOWER STEAMERS ❧ AROMATIC

	3–6 mo.	6–24 mo.	2–6 yr.	6+ yr.
Baking soda	1 cup	1 cup	1 cup	1 cup
Arrowroot powder or cornstarch	⅓ cup	⅓ cup	⅓ cup	⅓ cup
Water	⅓ cup + 2 tbsp.	⅓ cup + 2 tbsp.	⅓ cup + 2 tbsp.	⅓ cup + 2 tbsp.
Fir needle essential oil	1 drop	2 drops	2 drops	2 drops
Lemon essential oil	no drops	1 drop	1 drop	1 drop
Rosalina essential oil	2 drops	2 drops	2 drops	2 drops

1. Preheat oven to 350°F.
2. In a medium bowl, combine the baking soda, arrowroot powder, and water to make a thick paste.
3. Pour the mixture into a silicone muffin pan, filling each cup halfway.
4. Bake in the oven for 20 minutes. Allow to sit out overnight if extra dry time is needed.
5. Pop the steamers out of the molds, and store them in a wide-mouthed Mason jar.
6. To use, add the essential oils to one disc and place the disc at the opposite end of the shower, away from the water. Close the door to the bathroom and breathe in the steamy aromatherapy.

PNEUMONIA NIXER CHEST RUB
MAKES ABOUT 4 OUNCES ⇝ AROMATIC

	3–6 mo.	6–24 mo.	2–6 yr.	6+ yr.
Unrefined coconut oil	½ cup	½ cup	½ cup	½ cup
Fir needle essential oil	2 drops	10 drops	15 drops	20 drops
Lavender essential oil	1 drop	5 drops	10 drops	15 drops
Rosalina essential oil	1 drop	5 drops	10 drops	15 drops

1. In a small pan over low heat, melt the coconut oil.
2. Once melted, remove from heat, add the fir needle, lavender, and rosalina essential oils, and stir to combine.
3. Pour into a Mason jar, and put into the freezer for 20 minutes to harden.
4. Apply to the chest, back, neck, and the bottoms of feet. Cover the feet with socks after application. Store any unused rub in a cool, dark location.

Poison Ivy, Oak, and Sumac

If your family spends even a small amount of time outdoors, you're at risk for running into poison ivy, oak, and sumac. These poisonous plants cause extremely itchy, painful rashes. If your child comes in contact with one of these plants, antibacterial and anti-inflammatory essential oils such as lavender, tea tree, rosalina, geranium, chamomile, blue tansy, frankincense, spearmint, palmarosa, fir needle, cypress, juniper berry, pine, neroli, coriander, patchouli, marjoram, rose, and sandalwood can help to soothe the itch, reduce inflammation, and heal the sores.

SOOTHING ANTI-ITCH PASTE
MAKES ABOUT 3 OUNCES ➤ TOPICAL

	3–6 mo.	6–24 mo.	2–6 yr.	6+ yr.
Bentonite clay	3 tbsp.	3 tbsp.	3 tbsp.	3 tbsp.
Baking soda	2 tbsp.	2 tbsp.	2 tbsp.	2 tbsp.
Vegetable glycerin	1 tbsp.	1 tbsp.	1 tbsp.	1 tbsp.
Filtered water or witch hazel	enough to form a paste	enough to form a paste	enough to form a paste	enough to form a paste
Blue tansy essential oil	1 drop	5 drops	5 drops	5 drops
Lavender essential oil	3 drops	15 drops	15 drops	15 drops

1. Add all the ingredients to a Mason jar, and stir to combine.
2. Apply to rashes to relieve itchiness, pain, and inflammation. Store any unused paste in the refrigerator.

ITCH-B-GONE OAT BATH

MAKES 1 TREATMENT ⇾ TOPICAL

	3–6 mo.	6–24 mo.	2–6 yr.	6+ yr.
Oats, finely ground	1 cup	1 cup	1 cup	1 cup
Baking soda	¼ cup	¼ cup	¼ cup	¼ cup
German chamomile essential oil	1 drop	2 drops	3 drops	4 drops
Rosalina essential oil	1 drop	1 drop	3 drops	3 drops

1. Pulse the oats in a blender or food processor until powdered. Add in the baking soda, and pulse until the mixture is well blended.

2. Add the German chamomile and rosalina essential oils, and pulse a few times more to mix in.

3. To use, either add straight to the bath under running water, or add to a fine mesh bag or an old, clean sock, then toss it into the bathtub under the running water. Have your child soak in the tub at least 20 minutes. Follow the bath with an Anti-Itch Calamine Lotion (page 142). Store in a Mason jar in a cool, dry location, when not in use.

SOOTHE THE ITCH SALVE

MAKES ABOUT 4 OUNCES ⇾ TOPICAL

	3–6 mo.	6–24 mo.	2–6 yr.	6+ yr.
Unrefined coconut oil	¼ cup	¼ cup	¼ cup	¼ cup
Extra-virgin olive oil	2 tbsp.	2 tbsp.	2 tbsp.	2 tbsp.
Beeswax	2 tbsp.	2 tbsp.	2 tbsp.	2 tbsp.
German chamomile essential oil	1 drop	5 drops	7 drops	10 drops
Lavender essential oil	2 drops	5 drops	10 drops	15 drops
Rosalina essential oil	1 drop	5 drops	10 drops	15 drops

1. In a small pan over low heat, heat the coconut oil, olive oil, and beeswax.
2. Once melted, remove from heat, and add the German chamomile, lavender, and rosalina essential oils.
3. Pour into a Mason jar, and put into the freezer for 20 minutes to harden.
4. Apply the salve to itchy skin and rashes whenever needed. Store the salve in a cool, dark location.

AWESOME ADDITION Calendula and lavender are well known for their anti-inflammatory and skin-healing properties, and would make a great addition to this salve. Steep 2 tablespoons (total) of the herbs in the coconut oil over low heat for 2 hours. Strain before using in this recipe.

Ringworm

Contrary to its name, ringworm does not actually involve a worm; ringworm is caused by a fungal infection on the skin. The telltale signs of ringworm are a circular bull's eye with healthy skin in the middle. Ringworm is contagious and can be spread from direct contact with a personal or pet infected with the fungus. Soothing antifungal essential oils including lavender, tea tree, rosalina, coriander, sweet orange, lemon, mandarin, grapefruit, tangerine, geranium, chamomile, pine, cedarwood, and frankincense can all help combat and heal up ringworm.

RINGWORM REMOVER SALVE
MAKES ABOUT 4 OUNCES ⇒ TOPICAL

	3–6 mo.	6–24 mo.	2–6 yr.	6+ yr.
Unrefined coconut oil	¼ cup	¼ cup	¼ cup	¼ cup
Beeswax pastilles	2 tbsp.	2 tbsp.	2 tbsp.	2 tbsp.
Unrefined shea butter	2 tbsp.	2 tbsp.	2 tbsp.	2 tbsp.
Geranium essential oil	no drops	5 drops	10 drops	15 drops
Lavender essential oil	2 drops	10 drops	15 drops	20 drops
Tea tree essential oil	2 drops	5 drops	10 drops	15 drops

1. In a small pan over medium heat, melt the coconut oil, beeswax, and shea butter.
2. Once melted, remove from heat, and add the geranium, lavender, and tea tree essential oils.
3. Pour into a Mason jar, and put into the freezer for 20 minutes to harden.
4. Apply the salve to ringworm twice daily. Be persistent with the treatment because fungal infections can be difficult to get rid of if you aren't consistent. Store any unused salve in a cool, dark location.

AWESOME ADDITION Black walnut hulls and chaparral are well known for their antifungal properties and would make a great addition to this salve. Steep 2 tablespoons (total) of the herbs in the coconut oil over low heat for 2 hours. Strain before using in this recipe.

RINGWORM SCALP TREATMENT

MAKES 1 TREATMENT ❧ TOPICAL

	3–6 mo.	6–24 mo.	2–6 yr.	6+ yr.
Unrefined coconut oil	1 tbsp.	1 tbsp.	1 tbsp.	1 tbsp.
Lavender essential oil	1 drop	2 drops	4 drops	5 drops
Palmarosa essential oil	no drops	1 drop	2 drops	3 drops
Tea tree essential oil	no drops	2 drops	3 drops	5 drops
Aloe vera gel	1 tbsp.	1 tbsp.	1 tbsp.	1 tbsp.

1. In a small pan over low heat, melt the coconut oil, then add the lavender, palmarosa, and tea tree essential oils, stirring to combine.
2. While whisking the coconut oil mixture, slowly mix in the aloe vera gel.
3. Apply the treatment to your child's scalp, cover with plastic wrap or a shower cap, and let sit for 20 minutes before shampooing clean.

Sleep

While sleep is very important to a mama and her children, getting kids to go to sleep can be difficult. Any changes in the daily routine, illnesses, medications, or problems at school can cause sleep pattern disruptions. Essential oils that help to calm the body and ready the mind for sleep, aiding development of a natural sleep cycle, include lavender, chamomile, sweet orange, neroli, rosalina, vetiver, sandalwood, cedarwood, petitgrain, marjoram, vanilla, bergamot, clary sage, coriander, frankincense, lemon, mandarin, tangerine, valerian root, and ylang-ylang.

GOOD NIGHT SLEEP TIGHT AROMATHERAPY MASSAGE OIL

MAKES 1 OUNCE ⋗ TOPICAL ⋗ AROMATIC

	3–6 mo.	6–24 mo.	2–6 yr.	6+ yr.
Unrefined coconut oil	2 tbsp.	2 tbsp.	2 tbsp.	2 tbsp.
Lavender essential oil	1 drop	2 drops	3 drops	6 drops
Marjoram essential oil	no drops	1 drop	3 drops	6 drops
Sweet orange essential oil	1 drop	2 drops	3 drops	6 drops

1. In a small pan over low heat, melt the coconut oil.
2. Once melted, remove from heat, add the lavender, marjoram, and sweet orange essential oils, and stir to combine.
3. Pour into a Mason jar, and put into the freezer for 20 minutes to harden.
4. Apply a small amount to the child's chest, back of the neck, and feet before bedtime. Store any unused oil in a cool, dark location.

SWEET DREAMS DIFFUSER BLEND

MAKES ½ OUNCE ⋗ AROMATIC

1 teaspoon bergamot essential oil
1 teaspoon lavender essential oil

½ teaspoon Atlas cedarwood essential oil
½ teaspoon Roman chamomile essential oil

TO MAKE THE BLEND

Add all the essential oils to an empty essential oil bottle (or any dark glass bottle with a dropper), and gently swirl the bottle to combine. ➔

TO DIFFUSE THE BLEND

Add the recommended drops to a diffuser and diffuse throughout the room in 30-minute increments (30 minutes on/30 minutes off).

0–6 mo.	6–24 mo.	2–6 yr.	6+ yr.
2 drops	4 drops	6 drops	8 drops

RELAXING BEDTIME BUBBLE BATH
MAKES 1 TREATMENT ≫ TOPICAL ≫ AROMATIC

	3–6 mo.	6–24 mo.	2–6 yr.	6+ yr.
Lavender essential oil	2 drops	3 drops	5 drops	5 drops
Roman chamomile essential oil	no drops	1 drop	2 drops	2 drops
Tangerine essential oil	no drops	2 drops	3 drops	3 drops
Vanilla CO_2 (12%)	1 drop	1 drop	2 drops	2 drops
Unscented shampoo or castile soap	2 tbsp.	2 tbsp.	2 tbsp.	2 tbsp.
Epsom salt	1 cup	1 cup	1 cup	1 cup

1. In a small bowl, stir together the lavender, Roman chamomile, tangerine, and vanilla CO_2 essential oils with the shampoo or liquid soap.
2. Place the Epsom salt in a medium bowl and stir in the soap mixture.
3. Pour the mixture under the running bath water as you fill the tub.

Sneezing

Sneezing is your nose's defense against irritants, such as dust, pollen, and dander getting into the nasal passages. Sneezing can be a symptom of allergies, colds, the flu, and more. Essential oils can help stop sneezing attacks by cleansing the air of pollutants, soothing inflamed membranes, and reducing allergies. Anti-inflammatory and antihistamine essential oils such as lavender, rosalina, chamomile, blue tansy, fir needle, cypress, juniper berry, geranium, rose, and spearmint can all help reduce or stop excessive sneezing.

STOP YOUR SNEEZING DIFFUSER BLEND
MAKES ½ OUNCE ⇒ AROMATIC

1 teaspoon lavender essential oil

1 teaspoon rosalina essential oil

½ teaspoon blue tansy essential oil

½ teaspoon fir needle essential oil

TO MAKE THE BLEND

Add all the essential oils to an empty essential oil bottle (or any dark glass bottle with a dropper), and gently swirl the bottle to combine.

TO DIFFUSE THE BLEND

Add the recommended drops to a diffuser and diffuse throughout the room in 30-minute increments (30 minutes on/30 minutes off).

0–6 mo.	6–24 mo.	2–6 yr.	6+ yr.
2 drops	4 drops	6 drops	8 drops

STOP SNEEZING AROMATHERAPY INHALER

MAKES 1 TREATMENT ❧ AROMATIC

	3–6 mo.	6–24 mo.	2–6 yr.	6+ yr.
Blue tansy essential oil	1 drop	3 drops	5 drops	5 drops
Fir needle essential oil	1 drop	3 drops	5 drops	5 drops
German chamomile essential oil	1 drop	3 drops	5 drops	5 drops
Rosalina essential oil	1 drop	3 drops	5 drops	5 drops

1. Combine all the essential oils in a small glass bowl.
2. Using tweezers, add the wick (the cotton pad) of an aromatherapy personal inhaler to the bowl and roll it around until it's soaked up all of the essential oils mixture.
3. Use the tweezers to transfer the wick to the inhaler tube. Close the tube and label the inhaler.
4. Let your child take a whiff of the inhaler whenever sneezing won't quit.

Sniffles and Runny Nose

Everything from allergies, sinus infections, teething, colds, the flu, and even cold weather can cause your child to get a runny nose. Aromatherapy can help soothe the sniffles and even stop a runny nose in its tracks. Essential oils that help to open up the airways and soothe sinus passages include lavender, chamomile, marjoram, rosalina, fir needle, cypress, juniper berry, spruce, cedarwood, spearmint, lemon, blue tansy, tea tree, frankincense, and palmarosa.

SNIFFLES SNUFFER AROMATHERAPY INHALER

MAKES 1 TREATMENT ❧ AROMATIC

	3–6 mo.	6–24 mo.	2–6 yr.	6+ yr.
Blue tansy essential oil	1 drop	3 drops	5 drops	5 drops
Lavender essential oil	1 drop	3 drops	5 drops	5 drops
Lemon essential oil	1 drop	3 drops	5 drops	5 drops
Rosalina essential oil	1 drop	3 drops	5 drops	5 drops

1. Combine all the essential oils in a small glass bowl.
2. Using tweezers, add the wick (the cotton pad) of an aromatherapy personal inhaler to the bowl and roll it around until it's soaked up all of the essential oils mixture.
3. Use the tweezers to transfer the wick to the inhaler tube. Close the tube and label the inhaler.
4. Let your child take a whiff of the inhaler whenever needed.

STOP THE SNIFFLES DIFFUSER BLEND

MAKES ½ OUNCE ❧ AROMATIC

1 teaspoon fir needle essential oil
1 teaspoon rosalina essential oil

½ teaspoon cypress essential oil
½ teaspoon spearmint essential oil

TO MAKE THE BLEND

Add all the essential oils to an empty essential oil bottle (or any dark glass bottle with a dropper), and gently swirl the bottle to combine. ➜

Add the recommended drops to a diffuser and diffuse throughout the room in 30-minute increments (30 minutes on/30 minutes off).

0–6 mo.	6–24 mo.	2–6 yr.	6+ yr.
2 drops	4 drops	6 drops	8 drops

Sore Throat

A common occurrence in childhood, sore throats often lasts for 24 hours. If, however, your child has a sore throat for longer than 5 days and an accompanying fever, consult your medical practitioner to rule out anything serious. Essential oils including lavender, ginger, helichrysum, chamomile, marjoram, rosalina, tea tree, geranium, spearmint, frankincense, and lemon can help soothe the pain of the sore throat and stimulate the immune system to help your child heal faster. Hydrosols such as chamomile, lavender, tea tree, and peppermint can help soothe the pain internally when used with a gargle or throat spray.

SOOTHING SORE THROAT SPRAY
MAKES ABOUT 4 OUNCES » SAFE FOR AGES 1+ YEAR

¼ cup peppermint hydrosol
¼ cup chamomile hydrosol

2 tablespoons sage leaf
1 tablespoon raw unfiltered honey

1. In a small pan over low heat, heat the hydrosols.
2. Add the sage leaf and let steep for 15 minutes.
3. Strain and add the raw unfiltered honey, stirring until it dissolves.
4. Pour the mixture into a 4-ounce spray bottle, storing in the refrigerator when not in use.
5. To use, have your child open their mouth wide and spray into the back of their throat. Use whenever needed.

AWESOME ADDITION Echinacea root not only helps to boost the immune system to help you get over illness faster, it also provides a numbing action when used on skin or irritated membranes. To add to this recipe, add 1 tablespoon echinacea root to the sage leaf tea in step 2.

SORE THROAT AROMATHERAPY ROLL-ON
MAKES ⅓ OUNCE ❧ TOPICAL ❧ AROMATIC

	3–6 mo.	6–24 mo.	2–6 yr.	6+ yr.
Lavender essential oil	1 drop	2 drops	1 drop	2 drops
Rosalina essential oil	no drops	no drops	1 drop	2 drops
Spearmint essential oil	no drops	no drops	1 drop	2 drops
Fractionated coconut oil	to fill	to fill	to fill	to fill

1. Add the lavender, rosalina, and spearmint essential oils to a ⅓-ounce glass roll-on bottle.
2. Add enough fractionated coconut oil to fill the bottle. Place the roller ball and cap on and gently swirl to combine. Don't forget to label your creation.
3. To use, roll onto your child's neck, lymph nodes, and chest whenever needed.

Teething

A slight fever, extra drool, irritability, swollen gums, and loss of appetite are all symptoms that your baby may be cutting teeth. Although you'll see many DIY gels online recommending clove essential oil, it is *not* recommended for use on children under the age of 2 years as it can greatly irritate mucous membranes, especially those of young children and babies. In fact, anyone with hypersensitive, diseased, or damaged skin should avoid clove essential oil topically, and healthy adults are cautioned to use it at no greater than a dilution of 0.5 percent. If you have already used clove essential oil on your baby's gums, stop its use immediately.

JAWLINE MASSAGE OIL

MAKES ABOUT 1 OUNCE ❥ TOPICAL

	3–6 mo.	6–24 mo.	2–6 yr.	6+ yr.
Lavender essential oil	1 drop	2 drops	3 drops	6 drops
Roman chamomile essential oil	1 drop	2 drops	3 drops	6 drops
Fractionated coconut oil or similar carrier oil	2 tbsp.	2 tbsp.	2 tbsp.	2 tbsp.

1. Combine all the ingredients in a 1-ounce bottle. Gently swirl to combine.
2. Massage 2 drops onto the jawline and cheeks as needed.

SAFETY TIP This blend is for external use only.

CHAMOMILE GUM POPS

MAKES 4 OUNCES ICE POPS ➢ SAFE FOR AGES 6+ MONTHS

2 tablespoons chamomile hydrosol

¼ cup chamomile tea

2 tablespoons applesauce

1. Combine all the ingredients in a small bowl and pour into ice pop molds.
2. Freeze overnight.
3. Offer an ice pop to your child whenever discomfort arises.

SAFETY TIP These ice pops are not safe for babies and children under 6 months old.

Thrush

Thrush is a common type of yeast that can be found in many adults and children alike. It presents as diaper rashes in babies, a white rash inside the mouth, and even yeast infections in the vagina. Babies can catch it during labor from their mother's vagina, from infected nipples while feeding, or the overuse of antibiotics. The choice of treatment will depend upon the location of the fungal infection. Antifungal essential oils and hydrosols can be used in baby wipes, antifungal salves, and mouthwashes. These include essential oils of lavender, chamomile, spearmint, geranium, tea tree, rosalina, palmarosa, lemon, sweet orange, frankincense, neroli, petitgrain, blue tansy, and helichrysum.

ANTIFUNGAL WIPES

MAKES 24 WIPES ❧ TOPICAL

	3–6 mo.	6–24 mo.	2–6 yr.	6+ yr.
Unrefined coconut oil	1 tbsp.	1 tbsp.	1 tbsp.	1 tbsp.
Lavender essential oil	1 drop	3 drops	5 drops	5 drops
Tea tree essential oil	1 drop	3 drops	5 drops	5 drops
Witch hazel	½ cup	½ cup	½ cup	½ cup

1. In a small pan over low heat, melt the coconut oil. Add the lavender and tea tree essential oils and stir to combine.
2. In a medium glass bowl, whisk the witch hazel into the coconut oil mixture.
3. Cut 12 paper towels in half and stack them in a glass container with a lid. Pour the mixture over the paper towels. The paper towels should soak up all the liquid.
4. Cover the wipes with the lid and store in the refrigerator when not using for up to 1 month.

ANTIFUNGAL MOUTHWASH

MAKES 8 OUNCES ❧ SAFE FOR ALL AGES

½ cup peppermint hydrosol
¼ cup lavender hydrosol
¼ cup filtered water

1 tablespoon raw unfiltered honey (for infants under 1 year, substitute maple syrup or vegetable glycerin)

1. Combine all the ingredients in an 8-ounce jar or container. Shake until the honey is dissolved.
2. For children who can spit, have them gargle with this mouthwash before spitting out. For infants, use a cotton swab and gently apply.
3. Store any unused mouthwash in a cool, dark location.

Umbilical Cord Care

When your baby is born, the umbilical cord is clamped and cut, officially separating your child from your womb. Over the next 7 to 10 days the cord will shrivel up and eventually fall off, leaving your baby with their belly button. Gently wash and pat dry the stump daily. Do not apply any coconut oil or salves to the belly button until the stump falls off. Hydrosols are very gentle and much safer to use on newborns than essential oils. Beyond gentle cleansing, it is advised to let the stump heal on its own without any salves or creams.

ANTIBACTERIAL UMBILICAL CORD WASH

MAKES ABOUT 4 OUNCES ❧ TOPICAL

1 tablespoon aloe vera gel
¼ cup plus 1 tablespoon
  lavender hydrosol

2 tablespoons witch hazel

1. Combine the aloe vera gel, lavender hydrosol, and witch hazel in a 4-ounce spray bottle. Gently swirl the bottle to combine.
2. To use, spray onto the umbilical cord stump and gently pat dry with a clean cloth. Store any unused wash in a cool, dark location.

SUBSTITUTION TIP If you do not have lavender hydrosol on hand, chamomile or rose hydrosol are extremely gentle, and both contain anti-inflammatory properties that soothe inflamed skin and heal up infections. Either would make a great substitution for the lavender.

Warts

Warts, a symptom of the human papillomavirus (HPV), are benign skin growths contracted through physical contact or touching infected surfaces. There are several different types of warts including hand warts, plantar warts, flat warts, and genital warts. The essential oils of lavender, tea tree, geranium, lemon, marjoram, cypress, rosalina, and cedarwood can help to heal up and eliminate warts. The following remedies are for hand and foot warts only, not for facial or genital warts. Consult with your medical practitioner if warts last longer than 8 weeks, are swollen and red, or if a wart is bleeding.

WARTS-B-GONE OINTMENT
MAKES ABOUT 4 OUNCES ➤ TOPICAL

	3–6 mo.	6–24 mo.	2–6 yr.	6+ yr.
Unrefined coconut oil	¼ cup	¼ cup	¼ cup	¼ cup
Extra-virgin olive oil	2 tbsp.	2 tbsp.	2 tbsp.	2 tbsp.
Beeswax pastilles	2 tbsp.	2 tbsp.	2 tbsp.	2 tbsp.
Cypress essential oil	no drops	5 drops	10 drops	15 drops
Steam-distilled lemon essential oil	no drops	5 drops	10 drops	15 drops
Marjoram essential oil	no drops	10 drops	15 drops	20 drops

1. In a small pan over low heat, heat the coconut oil, olive oil, and beeswax.
2. Once the coconut oil and beeswax have melted, remove from the heat, and add the cypress, lemon, and marjoram essential oils.
3. Pour into a Mason jar, and put into the freezer for 20 minutes to harden.
4. Apply to the wart two times daily and cover with a bandage. Store the ointment in a cool, dark location.

NO MORE WARTS OIL

MAKES ABOUT 4 OUNCES ❧ TOPICAL

	3–6 mo.	6–24 mo.	2–6 yr.	6+ yr.
Unrefined coconut oil	½ cup	½ cup	½ cup	½ cup
Steam-distilled lemon essential oil	no drops	5 drops	10 drops	15 drops
Rosalina essential oil	4 drop	5 drops	10 drops	15 drops
Tea tree essential oil	no drops	10 drops	20 drops	30 drops

1. In a small pan over low heat, melt the coconut oil.
2. Once melted, remove from heat, add the lemon, rosalina, and tea tree essential oils, and stir to combine.
3. Pour into a Mason jar, and put into the freezer for 20 minutes to harden.
4. Apply to the wart two times daily and cover with a bandage. Store the oil in a cool, dark location.

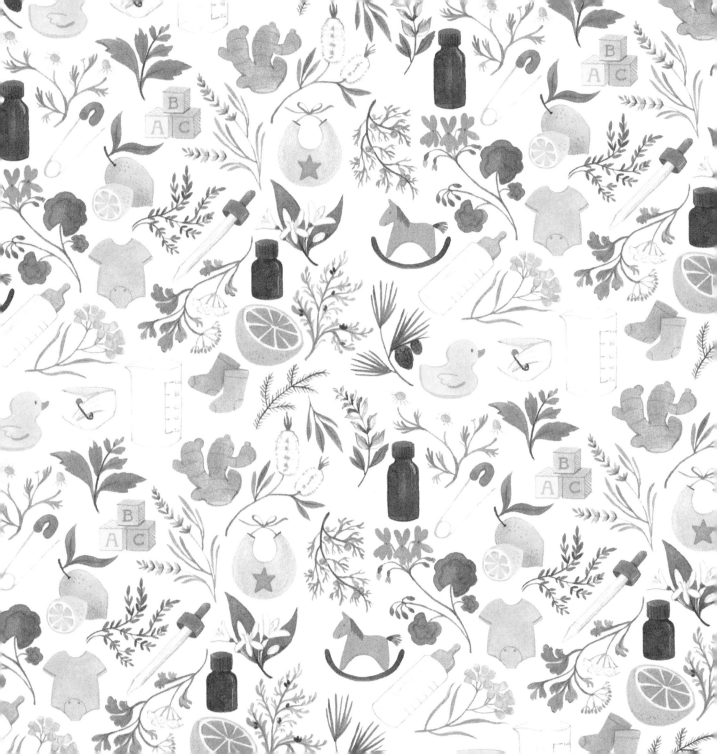

PART THREE

30 Family-Friendly Essential Oils to Know

There are hundreds of essential oils that can make hundreds, if not thousands, of healing blends, but there are only a relative handful of essential oils that can be used safely for everyday applications. Here, I'll give you 30 of the most useful. In each profile, I've included the oil's Latin name, as these can be helpful to know when you're shopping—not all essential oil companies call each oil by the same name, but the Latin name never changes.

As you delve further into your education on essential oils and their uses, it is important to become more familiar with individual oils and their many medicinal purposes and safety precautions. I suggest you start an essential oil profile notebook and begin learning about each essential oil individually and more in depth. Other books and the Internet can provide you with a plethora of information, but here you'll find a handy reference to the essential oils you're likely to find yourself buying and using for your family the most.

Bergamot

CITRUS BERGAMIA

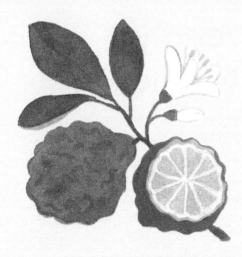

Bergamot essential oil is cold-pressed from the peel of the citrus fruit and has a fresh, sweet, and fruity scent. It has been used for centuries in Italian folk medicine, but is most commonly known for its use in perfumery and potpourri. Although the fruit itself is inedible, the essential oil has many uses, including in culinary flavoring and in household cleaning supplies. Recent research has shown bergamot to be particularly beneficial for healing skin, mouth, and respiratory infections.

BLENDS WELL WITH

chamomile, citrus oils, coriander, cypress, geranium, lavender

CAN BE SUBSTITUTED WITH

grapefruit, lemon, sweet orange

MEDICINAL PROPERTIES

analgesic, antidepressant, antiseptic, antispasmodic, carminative, febrifuge, stimulant, vulnerary

IDEAL FOR TREATING

anxiety, colds, eczema, fever, flu, psoriasis, sore throat, thrush, wounds, and for use as insect repellent

PRECAUTIONS

avoid sunlight after use (unless certified bergapten-free—bergapten is the chemical in bergamot essential oil that causes phototoxicity); avoid use of old or oxidized oils

Black Pepper

PIPER NIGRUM

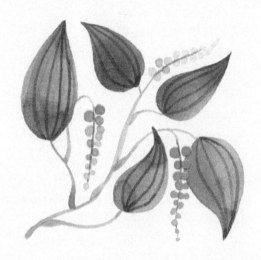

BLENDS WELL WITH

clary sage, frankincense, lavender, marjoram, sandalwood, sweet orange

CAN BE SUBSTITUTED WITH

bergamot, ginger, sandalwood

MEDICINAL PROPERTIES

analgesic, antimicrobial, antiseptic, antispasmodic, bactericidal, carminative, febrifuge, stimulant

IDEAL FOR TREATING

catarrh, colds, constipation, diarrhea, flu, heartburn, infections and viruses, muscular aches and pains, nausea

PRECAUTIONS

avoid use of old or oxidized oils

One of the oldest-known spices, with records of its use dating back to the ancient Greeks, Romans, and Egyptians, black pepper was used extensively in the Egyptian embalming process. The oil's scent is faintly reminiscent of freshly ground pepper, and great at relieving muscle pain, achy joints, and menstrual pains. Highly antiseptic, it is a good addition to a diffuser when illness strikes, killing airborne germs. Used for centuries in food, black pepper naturally helps with digestive problems and poor circulation.

Blue Tansy

TANACETUM ANNUUM

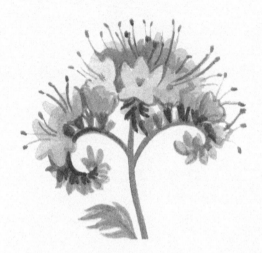

Often mistaken for German chamomile and tansy, this subtly apple-scented essential oil gets its name from its deep blue color. Blue tansy essential oil is nontoxic and safe for pregnant women and babies. Its telltale blue color comes from the chemical constituent, chamazulene, which also gives blue tansy its natural antihistamine properties. It's perfect for treating asthma, allergies, or sinusitis. Blue tansy is a gentle oil that can calm and soothe overstimulated children, giving mom a chance to relax.

BLENDS WELL WITH

chamomile, citrus oils, coriander, lavender, rosalina, spruce

CAN BE SUBSTITUTED WITH

chamomile (German), helichrysum, neroli

MEDICINAL PROPERTIES

analgesic, anti-allergenic, antihistamine, anti-inflammatory, antispasmodic, bactericidal, carminative, fungicidal, vulnerary

IDEAL FOR TREATING

asthma, allergies, colds, cuts, eczema, insect bites, muscle pain, stress and tension, wounds

PRECAUTIONS

none known

Cedarwood Atlas and Virginia

CEDRUS ATLANTICA, JUNIPERUS VIRGINIANA

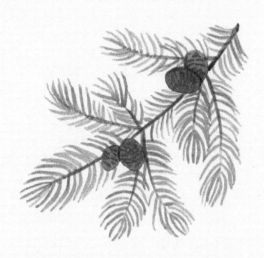

Cedarwood was used by the Greeks and Romans to cleanse and scent the air, while the ancient Egyptians used it in perfumes and embalming. Atlas cedarwood essential oil has been shown to help people with ADHD be calm and better focused and is perfect for people having trouble sleeping because of an over-active mind. Virginia cedarwood has a similar profile and is also a fantastic natural insect repellent, protecting your home and body from pesky bugs of all types.

BLENDS WELL WITH

bergamot, clary sage, cypress, lavender, neroli, palmarosa

CAN BE SUBSTITUTED WITH

cypress, fir needle

MEDICINAL PROPERTIES

antiseptic, astringent, diuretic, expectorant, fungicidal, mucolytic, sedative (nervous), stimulant (circulatory)

IDEAL FOR TREATING

arthritis, bronchitis, catarrh, congestion, cough, dandruff, eczema, fungal infections, hair loss, nervous tension and stress, and for use as insect repellent

PRECAUTIONS

none known

Chamomile German

MATRICARIA RECUTITA, MATRICARIA CHAMOMILLA

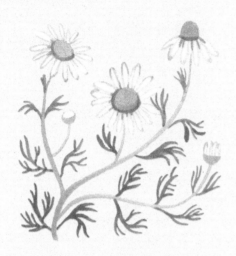

Well known for its skin-healing properties, German chamomile is very calming and soothing to the mind and body. Rich in chamazulene, German chamomile is blue in color and naturally powerful against allergies, infections, and wounds of all kinds. This light, floral-scented essential oil is great at calming children and even safe for the littlest babies at 3 months of age. Its natural anti-inflammatory properties make German chamomile soothing on sore muscles, and it can stop muscle spasms or cramps almost instantly. While very similar to Roman chamomile, German chamomile is better for skin and wound applications.

BLENDS WELL WITH

bergamot, citrus oils, clary sage, frankincense, lavender, marjoram

CAN BE SUBSTITUTED WITH

blue tansy, chamomile (Roman), lavender, neroli

MEDICINAL PROPERTIES

analgesic, anti-allergenic, anti-inflammatory, antispasmodic, bactericidal, carminative, fungicidal, vulnerary

IDEAL FOR TREATING

allergies, burns, cuts, dermatitis, eczema, headaches, insect bites, nausea, teething, wounds

PRECAUTIONS

avoid use if allergic to ragweed

Chamomile Roman

ANTHEMIS NOBILIS

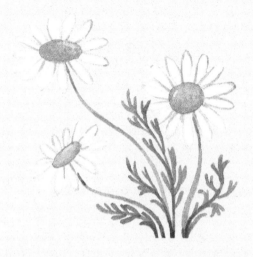

BLENDS WELL WITH

bergamot, clary sage, geranium, lavender, neroli, palmarosa

CAN BE SUBSTITUTED WITH

chamomile (German), lavender, neroli

MEDICINAL PROPERTIES

analgesic, antineuralgic, antiseptic, antispasmodic, bactericidal, carminative, febrifuge, vulnerary

IDEAL FOR TREATING

headaches, insomnia, indigestion, muscular pain, nausea, neuralgia, sprains, stress, teething, wounds

PRECAUTIONS

avoid use if allergic to ragweed

This apple-scented essential oil is one of the gentlest of the bunch. While very similar to German chamomile, Roman chamomile is more effective at calming the mind and soothing upset stomachs. It's great for helping little ones drift off to sleep but can also calm a toddler meltdown almost instantly. Naturally anti-inflammatory, Roman chamomile helps soothe overworked muscles as well as overworked minds.

Cinnamon Leaf

CINNAMOMUM ZEYLANICUM, CINNAMOMUM VERUM

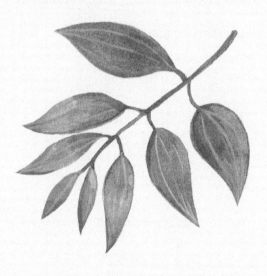

The utterly recognizable warm and inviting aroma of cinnamon has been enticing humans for centuries. Cinnamon leaf essential oil is the only cinnamon that should be used topically, unlike cinnamon bark, which should only be diffused. Extremely antiseptic, antibacterial, and antiviral, diffused cinnamon leaf essential oil kills airborne cold and flu germs. It also helps to stimulate the immune system, boosting your body's ability to fight off infection. Cinnamon bark essential oil should be avoided in all dermal applications because it is very irritating and known to cause sensitization.

BLENDS WELL WITH

citrus oils, clove, fir needle, frankincense, ginger, vanilla

CAN BE SUBSTITUTED WITH

cinnamon bark (inhalation only), clove, ginger

MEDICINAL PROPERTIES

antimicrobial, antiseptic, antispasmodic

IDEAL FOR TREATING

circulation, colds, flu, indigestion, lice, menstrual pain, muscle pain, rheumatism, warts, and for killing germs

PRECAUTIONS

avoid use if pregnant; avoid topical use with children under 6 months old; maximum dermal use—no more than 0.5% (5 drops per ounce of carrier oil); may cause irritation

Clary Sage

SALVIA SCLAREA

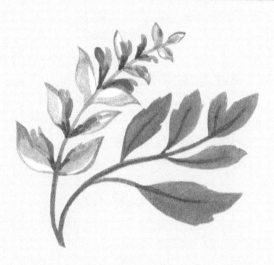

While not suggested for use during pregnancy, clary sage is helpful for most other types of common health issues for women, including problems with menstrual cycles, as well as during labor and delivery. This essential oil has been known to help enhance and strengthen contractions during labor, speeding things up when they have stalled out. Clary sage is one of the best oils for calming upset children and stressed-out mothers.

BLENDS WELL WITH

bergamot, black pepper, chamomile, citrus, lavender, patchouli

CAN BE SUBSTITUTED WITH

frankincense, lavender, sandalwood

MEDICINAL PROPERTIES

antidepressant, antiseptic, antispasmodic, astringent, carminative, emmenagogue, nervine, sedative

IDEAL FOR TREATING

asthma, cramps, dandruff, depression, flatulence, hair loss, labor pain, muscular aches and pains, nervous tension and stress, whooping cough

PRECAUTIONS

avoid use if pregnant; maximum dermal use—no more than 0.25% (2 drops per ounce of carrier oil); may cause irritation

Copaiba Balsam

COPAIFERA OFFICINALIS

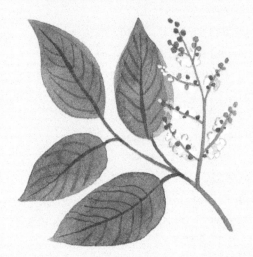

Used for centuries in Europe to treat bronchitis, Copaiba balsam is also widely known for its ability to reduce and heal inflammation from hemorrhoids. This delicate oil makes a great addition to any children's respiratory salve, because of its gentle nature and ability to get rid of mucus. If run in the diffuser, Copaiba balsam will kill airborne bacteria and fungus. This sweet-and-woody-scented essential oil is excellent at relieving pain, and makes a wonderful addition to any muscle or joint salve.

BLENDS WELL WITH

cedarwood, citrus oils, clary sage, rose, vanilla, ylang-ylang

CAN BE SUBSTITUTED WITH

cedarwood (Virginia), cypress, frankincense

MEDICINAL PROPERTIES

antifungal, anti-inflammatory, bactericidal, cicatrisant, disinfectant, diuretic, expectorant, stimulant

IDEAL FOR TREATING

bronchitis, colds, coughs, hemorrhoids, intestinal infections, muscle pain, stress

PRECAUTIONS

none known

Coriander

CORIANDRUM SATIVUM

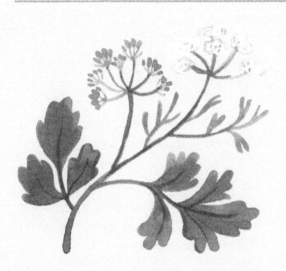

Derived from the seeds of cilantro, coriander essential oil has a delightful citrus scent that blends well with most essential oils. With a long history of use dating back to Ramses II, coriander is most widely known for healing digestive problems. Naturally good at relieving pain and stopping spasms, coriander essential oil is often used to treat muscle pains, arthritis, and even gout.

BLENDS WELL WITH

black pepper, cinnamon, citrus oils, frankincense, ginger, neroli

CAN BE SUBSTITUTED WITH

bergamot, lavender, ylang-ylang

MEDICINAL PROPERTIES

analgesic, anti-rheumatic, antispasmodic, bactericidal, carminative, digestive, fungicidal, stimulant

IDEAL FOR TREATING

arthritis, circulation, colds, flu, hemorrhoids, infections, migraine, muscular pain, nausea, neuralgia

PRECAUTIONS

none known

Cypress

CUPRESSUS SEMPERVIRENS

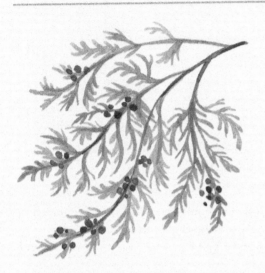

One thing comes to mind when smelling cypress essential oil—the woods. This forest in a bottle is used to support the respiratory system, clearing congestion and soothing incessant coughs. A great substitute for eucalyptus in a diffuser, cypress essential oil is much safer to use around young children and babies. It is well known for its ability to dilate blood vessels and tighten skin, and is often used to treat varicose veins, cellulite, and wrinkles.

BLENDS WELL WITH

black pepper, cedarwood, chamomile, citrus oils, ginger, pine

CAN BE SUBSTITUTED WITH

fir needle, juniper berry, pine

MEDICINAL PROPERTIES

antibacterial, anti-inflammatory, antiseptic, antispasmodic, astringent, febrifuge, styptic, vasoconstrictive

IDEAL FOR TREATING

asthma, cellulitis, colds, congestion, coughs, hemorrhoids, menstrual pain, muscle pain, varicose veins, whooping cough

PRECAUTIONS

avoid use of old or oxidized oils

Fir Needle

ABIES SIBIRICA

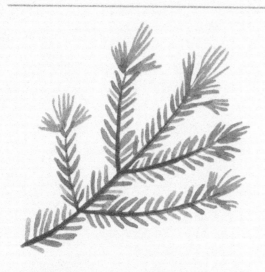

BLENDS WELL WITH

cinnamon, citrus oils, lavender, marjoram, pine, rosalina

CAN BE SUBSTITUTED WITH

cypress, juniper berry, pine

MEDICINAL PROPERTIES

analgesic, antiseptic, antitussive, astringent, expectorant, rubefacient, stimulant, tonic

IDEAL FOR TREATING

allergies, arthritis, bronchitis, catarrhal, coughs, colds, congestion, flu, muscle pain, sinusitis

PRECAUTIONS

avoid use of old or oxidized oils

One whiff of fir needle essential oil will have you dreaming you are among evergeens, their fallen needles covering the ground. This woodsy essential oil is wonderful for respiratory issues, helping to stop incessant coughing and get rid of mucus. Naturally antiseptic, fir needle used to be burned to cleanse the air of germs during and after childbirth. Gentle enough to use around babies and small children, fir needle is often used as a safe substitute for eucalyptus (which should be avoided with kids under age six).

Frankincense

BOSWELLIA CARTERI

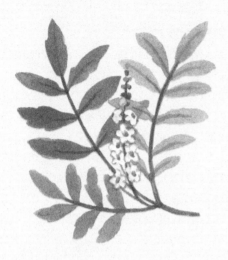

Used for thousands of years in incense and perfume, frankincense works well to heal bruising, swelling, and pain from traumatic injuries. This essential oil also banishes wrinkles and fine lines, helping to reduce visible signs of aging if used in anti-aging serums and creams. Frankincense is also highly antiseptic and when diffused, cleanses the air in the room and helps to support the immune system, shortening the time you or your baby is sick.

BLENDS WELL WITH
cinnamon, citrus oils, cypress, lavender, palmarosa, pine

CAN BE SUBSTITUTED WITH
cedarwood, lavender, sandalwood

MEDICINAL PROPERTIES
anti-inflammatory, antiseptic, astringent, carminative, emmenagogue, expectorant, sedative, vulnerary

IDEAL FOR TREATING
acne, asthma, bronchitis, catarrh, colds, flu, scars, stress and tension, wounds, wrinkles

PRECAUTIONS
avoid use of old or oxidized oils

Geranium

PELARGONIUM GRAVEOLENS

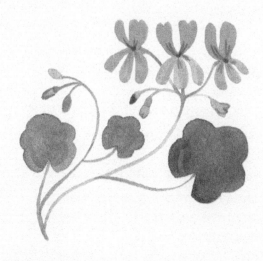

Sweet-smelling geranium essential oil invokes the childhood feeling of running free through a field of beautiful flowers. This florally scented essential oil is one of the best for treating nearly any skin condition you might face, soothing acne and other mild skin conditions, including cuts, scrapes, and other wounds. Geranium is beneficial for women's reproductive issues, including menstrual pains. Add the appropriate number of drops to a carrier oil and massage into the abdomen and lower back to relieve pain, bloating, and frazzled nerves.

BLENDS WELL WITH

chamomile, citrus oils, cypress, ginger, palmarosa, patchouli

CAN BE SUBSTITUTED WITH

frankincense, lavender, rose, ylang-ylang

MEDICINAL PROPERTIES

antidepressant, antihemorrhagic, anti-inflammatory, antiseptic, fungicidal, stimulant, styptic, vulnerary

IDEAL FOR TREATING

acne, breast engorgement, bruises, hemorrhoids, lice, ringworm, sore throat, stress and tension, wounds, and for use as insect repellent

PRECAUTIONS

maximum dermal use—no more than 17.5% (105 drops per 1 ounce carrier oil)

Ginger

ZINGIBER OFFICINALIS

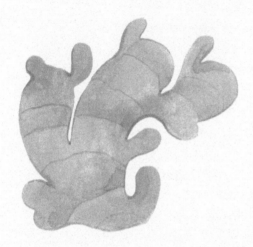

Spicy and warm, ginger is a powerhouse herb that has been used medicinally for centuries and is currently under study for its many benefits. Traditionally used for digestive issues, ginger essential oil is capable of easing nausea, flatulence, and even menstrual discomfort. When added to a carrier oil, ginger essential oil's warming sensation helps to soothe sore muscles and achy joints, naturally relieving the pain. Ginger essential oil also helps break up mucus, making it a great addition to any cough and congestion salve.

BLENDS WELL WITH

cedarwood, citrus oils, coriander, frankincense, geranium, palmarosa

CAN BE SUBSTITUTED WITH

cardamom, cinnamon, turmeric

MEDICINAL PROPERTIES

analgesic, antiseptic, antispasmodic, antitussive, bactericidal, carminative, expectorant, febrifuge

IDEAL FOR TREATING

arthritis, catarrh, circulation, colds, congestion, coughs, flatulence, flu, menstrual pain, muscle pain, nausea

PRECAUTIONS

maximum dermal use—no more than 1% (9 drops per ounce of carrier oil)

Grapefruit

CITRUS X PARADISI

Grapefruit essential oil's joyful scent helps to relieve depression and brighten the mood of any room. This upbeat oil is used in many different bath and body applications, but it shines in products made to get rid of cellulite and varicose veins. Naturally antibacterial and antiseptic, grapefruit essential oil cleanses the air of germs when diffused, and supports the immune system, keeping you healthy. This essential oil can cause a phototoxic reaction in the sun, if applied over the suggested maximum dermal use.

BLENDS WELL WITH

citrus oils, clary sage, frankincense, geranium, ginger, lavender

CAN BE SUBSTITUTED WITH

coriander, mandarin, sweet orange

MEDICINAL PROPERTIES

antibacterial, antidepressant, antiseptic, astringent, bactericidal, digestive, disinfectant, stimulant

IDEAL FOR TREATING

anxiety, cellulite, colds, depression, exhaustion, flu, hair loss, headaches, and for immune support

PRECAUTIONS

avoid sunlight after use (if applied over maximum dermal use); maximum dermal use—no more than 4% (36 drops per ounce of carrier oil); avoid use of old or oxidized oils

Helichrysum

HELICHRYSUM ITALICUM

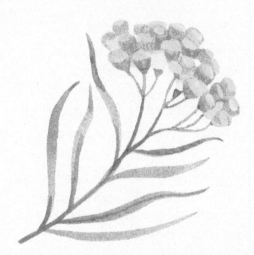

Known to many as *Immortelle*, helichrysum essential oil is known for its skin-healing and age-defying properties, helping care for acne, scars, wounds, and even wrinkles. Skin-care isn't the only place that this oil shines, though; its natural anti-inflammatory properties soothe achy muscles and joints, and it can calm a cough almost instantly. Naturally antiseptic and anti-allergenic, helichrysum essential oil does double duty in a diffuser, killing germs and easing allergens in the air.

BLENDS WELL WITH
chamomile, citrus oils, cypress, geranium, lavender, ylang-ylang

CAN BE SUBSTITUTED WITH
frankincense, lavender, sandalwood

MEDICINAL PROPERTIES
anti-allergenic, anti-inflammatory, antimicrobial, antitussive, antiseptic, expectorant, fungicidal, nervine

IDEAL FOR TREATING
acne, allergies, asthma, bronchitis, colds, cough, eczema, flu, muscle pain, wounds

PRECAUTIONS
none known

Lavender

LAVANDULA ANGUSTIFOLIA

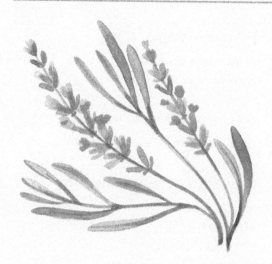

BLENDS WELL WITH

cedarwood, chamomile, citrus oils, coriander, fir needle, marjoram

CAN BE SUBSTITUTED WITH

chamomile, coriander, marjoram

MEDICINAL PROPERTIES

analgesic, anticonvulsive, antidepressant, antifungal, anti-inflammatory, antimicrobial, antiseptic, antispasmodic, antiviral, carminative, sedative, vulnerary

IDEAL FOR TREATING

burns, coughs, colds, dermatitis, eczema, flu, headaches, muscle pain, stress and tension, wounds

PRECAUTIONS

none known

One of the most versatile essential oils out there, lavender can do almost any job that calls for an essential oil. Highly antibacterial, antiseptic, antiviral, and antifungal, but still so gentle it can be used on babies, lavender rivals tea tree oil in its efficacy on wounds and versatility. Renowned for its ability to calm a restless mind and soothe tired achy muscles, lavender is most often used to aid sleep and relieve pain but can also help to calm overstimulated little ones. It can help healing and prevent scarring of all types when added to a carrier oil and applied to burns, cuts, and scrapes.

Lemon

CITRUS LIMON

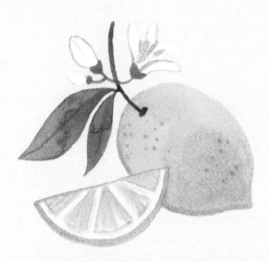

One of the most widely recognized scents in the world, lemon essential oil smells of freshly picked lemons. Naturally antiseptic and antimicrobial, lemon can be used in homemade cleaning products and even diffused in the air to kill germs throughout the home. This essential oil can cause a phototoxic reaction in the sun, if applied over the suggested maximum dermal use, however steam-distilled lemon essential oil does not contain the phototoxic properties that its cold-pressed counterpart does, and is thus suggested for skin-care use.

BLENDS WELL WITH

cedarwood, citrus oils, fir needle, frankincense, lavender, neroli

CAN BE SUBSTITUTED WITH

bergamot, sweet orange, tangerine

MEDICINAL PROPERTIES

antimicrobial, antispasmodic, antiseptic, astringent, bactericidal, carminative, febrifuge, insecticidal

IDEAL FOR TREATING

acne, asthma, cellulitis, circulation, colds, fevers, flu, scars, varicose veins, warts

PRECAUTIONS

avoid sunlight after use (if applied over maximum dermal use); maximum dermal use—no more than 2% if expressed (18 drops per ounce of carrier oil); avoid use of old or oxidized oils

Marjoram

ORIGANUM MAJORANA

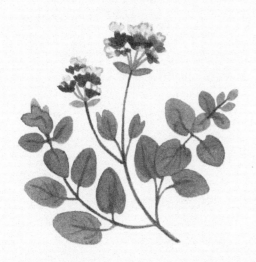

Well known in the culinary world, marjoram has also been used for centuries in herbal medicine. Much like the herb, this calming essential oil is exceptional at soothing achy muscles, spastic coughs, and even headaches. When combined with lavender essential oil in a carrier, the two can do no wrong, relieving pains and spasms and soothing little ones to sleep. This gentle essential oil is naturally antiseptic, antiviral, and bactericidal, making it a perfect addition to any kid-friendly, germ-killing diffuser blend.

BLENDS WELL WITH

cedarwood, chamomile, citrus oils, lavender, rosalina, tea tree

CAN BE SUBSTITUTED WITH

fir needle, ginger, lavender

MEDICINAL PROPERTIES

analgesic, antiseptic, antispasmodic, antiviral, bactericidal, carminative, expectorant, fungicidal, sedative, vulnerary

IDEAL FOR TREATING

asthma, bronchitis, bruises, colds, congestion, cough, flatulence, flu, headaches, muscle pain, stress and tension

PRECAUTIONS

none known

Neroli

CITRUS X AURANTIUM

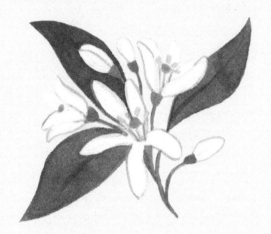

One of three essential oils deriving from the orange tree, neroli essential oil is made from the orange blossoms. This sweet and delicate floral essential oil naturally brightens the mood of any room, making it great for people experiencing grief, depression, or nervous tension. Neroli oil is also used in many skin-care products because it promotes a healthy complexion, and reduces fine lines and wrinkles.

BLENDS WELL WITH

chamomile, citrus oils, coriander, frankincense, ginger, lavender

CAN BE SUBSTITUTED WITH

bergamot, geranium, lavender

MEDICINAL PROPERTIES

antidepressant, antiseptic, antispasmodic, bactericidal, carminative, digestive, fungicidal, stimulant

IDEAL FOR TREATING

anxiety, circulation, depression, flatulence, scars, shock, stress and tension, stretch marks, thread veins, wrinkles

PRECAUTIONS

none known

Patchouli

POGOSTEMON CABLIN

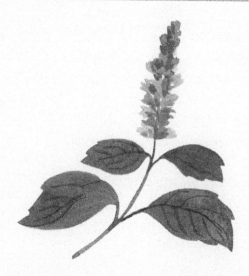

Known for its popularity with hippies, patchouli essential oil has become something of a punchline, but this earthy-scented essential oil is capable of a lot. Well known for its skin-healing abilities, patchouli essential oil can help reduce the appearance of fine lines, wrinkles, scars, and even stretch marks. Naturally antifungal, patchouli can also help heal up athlete's foot, ringworm, and other fungal infections. When diffused, it can help to ease nervous tension, increase focus, and even repel insects.

BLENDS WELL WITH

cedarwood, chamomile, citrus oils, coriander, lavender, sandalwood

CAN BE SUBSTITUTED WITH

frankincense, geranium, lavender

MEDICINAL PROPERTIES

antidepressant, anti-inflammatory, antimicrobial, antiseptic, antiviral, bactericidal, carminative, febrifuge, fungicidal

IDEAL FOR TREATING

acne, athlete's foot, colds, dermatitis, eczema, fevers, flu, fungal infections, stress, wounds, wrinkles, and for use as insect repellent

PRECAUTIONS

none known

Petitgrain

CITRUS X AURANTIUM

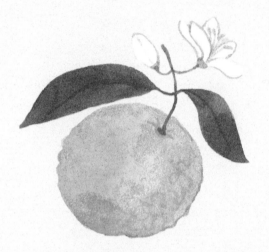

One of three essential oils that comes from the orange tree, petitgrain essential oil is made from the leaves and twigs. This soothing and uplifting essential oil can help alleviate depression, stress, and anxiety. When combined with lavender essential oil, petitgrain helps to quiet the mind so you can fall asleep faster. Because it is naturally antiseptic, it is great with acne and other skin-healing applications.

BLENDS WELL WITH

cedarwood, citrus oils, clary sage, frankincense, lavender, marjoram

CAN BE SUBSTITUTED WITH

bergamot, neroli, sweet orange

MEDICINAL PROPERTIES

antidepressant, antiseptic, antispasmodic, digestive, nervine, sedative, stimulant (digestive), stomachic, tonic

IDEAL FOR TREATING

acne, excessive perspiration, flatulence, hair loss, insomnia, stress

PRECAUTIONS

none known

Pine

PINUS SYLVESTRIS

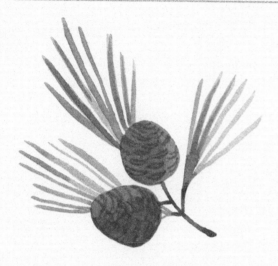

Well known for its ability to treat respiratory issues, pine essential oil is a much gentler option than eucalyptus in kid-safe vapor rub blends. Because of its natural ability to rid the lungs of mucus, it is effective when diffused for congestion, coughs, and sinusitis. Pine also kills germs and reduces allergens when diffused throughout your home—the reason it's added to cleaning products.

BLENDS WELL WITH

cedarwood, citronella, citrus oils, clary sage, frankincense, spruce

CAN BE SUBSTITUTED WITH

cypress, fir needle, spruce

MEDICINAL PROPERTIES

antimicrobial, antineuralgic, antiseptic, antiviral, bactericidal, expectorant, rubefacient, stimulant

IDEAL FOR TREATING

asthma, bronchitis, catarrh, circulation, colds, congestion, cough, flu, fatigue, lice, muscle pain

PRECAUTIONS

avoid use of old or oxidized oils

Rosalina

MELALEUCA ERICIFOLIA

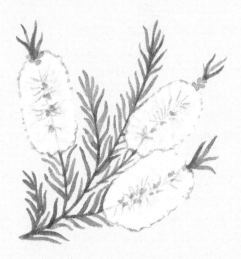

Known as "lavender tea tree" in Australia, rosalina essential oil is not as well known as either lavender or tea tree, but it definitely should be. Extremely gentle, this essential oil is the perfect substitute for eucalyptus in any kid-friendly vapor rub or diffuser blend. It works hard to help ease seasonal discomfort, calm coughs, and open up airways for better breathing. Carrying many of the same properties as lavender and tea tree, rosalina is great at cleansing and healing open wounds, dermatitis, and even acne.

BLENDS WELL WITH

blue tansy, citrus oils, coriander, fir needle, lavender, palmarosa, tea tree

CAN BE SUBSTITUTED WITH

lavender, marjoram, tea tree

MEDICINAL PROPERTIES

analgesic, antibacterial, antiseptic, antispasmodic, antiviral, anti-inflammatory, expectorant, febrifuge, mucolytic, sedative

IDEAL FOR TREATING

asthma, allergies, catarrh, circulation, colds, cough, congestion, fever, flu, insomnia, muscle pain, stress and tension

PRECAUTIONS

none known

Sandalwood Australian

SANTALUM SPICATUM

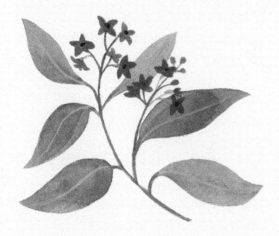

Used in traditional medicine for centuries in Australia, sandalwood is prized for its ability to relax the mind and ease tension. This slightly sweet, woody-smelling essential oil helps people shut down the mind before bed or while meditating. Australian sandalwood is the ecologically responsible choice over the endangered Indian sandalwood. Sandalwood is also used in skin-care products, effective at healing acne, scars, and even reducing the signs of fine lines and wrinkles.

BLENDS WELL WITH

cedarwood, chamomile, citrus oils, frankincense, lavender, patchouli

CAN BE SUBSTITUTED WITH

black pepper, clary sage, frankincense, helichrysum

MEDICINAL PROPERTIES

antidepressant, antiseptic, antispasmodic, bactericidal, carminative, expectorant, fungicidal, insecticidal, sedative

IDEAL FOR TREATING

acne, bronchitis, catarrh, colds, coughs, depression, flu, insomnia, nausea, muscle pain

PRECAUTIONS

none known

Spearmint

MENTHA SPICATA

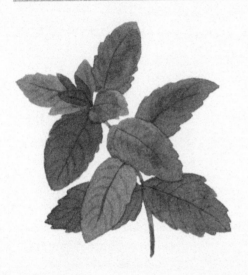

Aromatically sweet and minty, spearmint essential oil is the gentle younger brother of peppermint. Because it contains less menthol than peppermint but still has many of the same properties and uses, spearmint often replaces peppermint in applications for pregnant women and young children. When diluted in a carrier oil and applied topically to the abdomen, it can relieve nausea and bloating. When diffused, it reduces stress and anxiety while also improving focus and concentration.

BLENDS WELL WITH

citrus oils, lavender, marjoram, rosalina, vanilla

CAN BE SUBSTITUTED WITH

ginger, grapefruit, rosalina

MEDICINAL PROPERTIES

anesthetic, analgesic, antiseptic, antispasmodic, carminative, decongestant, expectorant, febrifuge, nervine, stimulant

IDEAL FOR TREATING

acne, asthma, colds, congestion, dermatitis, fevers, flu, flatulence, headache, nausea, vomiting

PRECAUTIONS

maximum dermal use—no more than 1.7% (16 drops per ounce of carrier oil)

Sweet Orange

CITRUS SINENSIS

Derived from the peel of the sweet orange fruit, this essential oil has a light and zesty citrus scent. While many other citrus essential oils are phototoxic, sweet orange essential oil typically is not. Sweet orange essential oil is used extensively in home and garden products because it contains 90% limonene, a constituent used in many natural household cleaners and insecticides. Sweet orange is gentle enough to be used with babies, but tough enough to effectively combat germs when your family gets a cold or the flu.

BLENDS WELL WITH

cedarwood, chamomile, cinnamon, citrus oils, coriander, frankincense, ginger, lavender

CAN BE SUBSTITUTED WITH

grapefruit, mandarin, tangerine

MEDICINAL PROPERTIES

antibacterial, antidepressant, anti-inflammatory, antiseptic, antispasmodic, bactericidal, carminative, digestive, expectorant, fungicidal, sedative

IDEAL FOR TREATING

acne, anxiety, cellulite, colds, congestion, cough, flu, insomnia, muscle spasms, nausea, stress

PRECAUTIONS

avoid use of old or oxidized oils

Tea Tree

MELALEUCA ALTERNIFOLIA

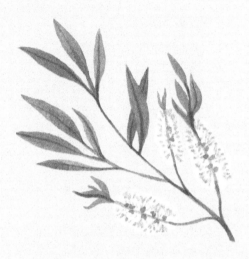

One of the most widely known and used essential oils in the world, tea tree is the go-to skin healer when it comes to cuts, infections, and fungi. Tea tree is an excellent fungicide, and will help clean out fungus and mold in bathrooms, kitchens, and even on plants in the garden when added to the watering can. Naturally antiseptic and extremely cleansing, diffused tea tree kills airborne germs and allergens. It is often used as a popular ingredient in natural acne care products because it cleanses the infection while soothing inflamed skin.

BLENDS WELL WITH

cedarwood, chamomile, citrus oils, lavender, marjoram, petitgrain

CAN BE SUBSTITUTED WITH

geranium, lavender, marjoram

MEDICINAL PROPERTIES

anti-infectious, anti-inflammatory, antiseptic, antiviral, bactericidal, expectorant, fungicidal, immuno-stimulant, vulnerary

IDEAL FOR TREATING

acne, asthma, athlete's foot, bronchitis, burns, catarrh, chicken pox, colds, cold sores, congestion, cough, fever, flu, thrush, wounds

PRECAUTIONS

maximum dermal use—no more than 15% (90 drops per ounce of carrier oil); avoid use of old or oxidized oils

Ylang-Ylang

CANANGA ODORATA

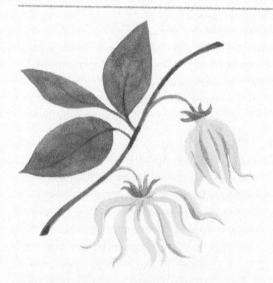

A flower from the tropical South Pacific, ylang-ylang essential oil smells intensely of the sweet, heady plant it's distilled from, so a little goes a long way, or you may get overpowered by the scent. Used in a diffuser, ylang-ylang can uplift the mood in a room and calm the mind if you're stressed. Added to a carrier oil, ylang-ylang makes a wonderful romantic massage oil.

BLENDS WELL WITH

chamomile, citrus oils, ginger, palmarosa, petitgrain, rose

CAN BE SUBSTITUTED WITH

geranium, lavender, neroli

MEDICINAL PROPERTIES

antibacterial, antidepressant, antifungal, anti-infectious, anti-inflammatory, antiseptic, hypotensive, nervine, sedative

IDEAL FOR TREATING

acne, anxiety, depression, hair loss, high blood pressure, insomnia, muscle spasms, stress and tension, and for use in skin-care

PRECAUTIONS

avoid topical use with children under 2 years of age; avoid topical use with hypersensitive, diseased, or damaged skin; maximum dermal use—no more than 0.8% (7 drops per ounce of carrier oil)

Essential Oils Labor Kit

Whether it's a home birth or a hospital birth, every woman needs a basic essential oils labor kit to tackle whatever comes her way.

CLARY SAGE   Though it is contraindicated during pregnancy, clary sage essential oil is a must-have during labor. It encourages and strengthens contractions, relieves muscular pain, and eases stress and anxiety.

GRAPEFRUIT   This refreshing and uplifting essential oil is not only antibacterial and antiseptic, but also raises spirits while calming nervous fears and anxiety. Grapefruit essential oil can help with nausea and vomiting during labor as well.

LAVENDER   This multifaceted essential oil can be used during nearly every stage of labor to ease pain and calm nervous fears. Lavender essential oil is naturally antiseptic and antibacterial and can be used to kill germs on hands and in the air.

ROMAN CHAMOMILE   Calming and soothing, chamomile essential oil is not just an anti-inflammatory, but also a natural digestive and can help with nausea during labor. This happy essential oil mixes well with grapefruit essential oil and can help lift the mood in the room when things get tense.

ROSALINA   Gentle and multifaceted like lavender, this cleansing essential oil is naturally antibacterial and antiseptic. Used as a gentle substitute for eucalyptus, when diffused, rosalina cleanses the air and can support healthy breathing. Also used as a natural pain reliever, diluting rosalina in a carrier oil and massaging onto the belly and back helps ease some of the labor pain.

SPEARMINT   The gentler version of peppermint, spearmint is great to keep on hand for any nausea or vomiting during labor. When diffused, this uplifting, happy essential oil reduces stress and anxiety while improving focus.

Ailments and Oils Quick-Reference Guide

Pregnancy

AILMENT	SUGGESTED ESSENTIAL OILS	METHODS OF APPLICATION
ACNE	Cedarwood, chamomile, geranium, lavender, palmarosa, rosalina, sweet orange, tea tree	STEAM, TOPICAL
ALLERGIES (HAY FEVER)	Blue tansy, chamomile (German), cypress, fir needle, frankincense, lavender, lemon, rosalina, sweet orange	INHALATION, STEAM
ANXIETY	Bergamot, cedarwood, chamomile, coriander, grapefruit, lavender, lemon, neroli, sandalwood, sweet orange, vanilla, ylang-ylang	INHALATION, ROOM SPRAY, TOPICAL
BACKACHES	Black pepper, cypress, fir needle, helichrysum, juniper, lavender, marjoram, rosalina, spearmint	BATH, TOPICAL
BREAST TENDERNESS	Chamomile, cypress, frankincense, geranium, grapefruit, helichrysum, lavender, marjoram, rosalina, ylang-ylang	MASSAGE, TOPICAL
CARPAL TUNNEL SYNDROME	Cypress, frankincense, ginger, helichrysum, lavender, marjoram, rosalina, spearmint, turmeric CO_2	MASSAGE, TOPICAL
CONSTIPATION	Chamomile, dill weed, frankincense, ginger, lemon, petitgrain, spearmint, sweet orange	MASSAGE, TOPICAL
COLD AND FLU	Blue tansy, chamomile, citrus, cypress, fir needle, frankincense, juniper, lavender, marjoram, palmarosa, pine, rosalina, spearmint, spruce, tea tree	BATH, COMPRESS, INHALATION,

→

AILMENT	SUGGESTED ESSENTIAL OILS	METHODS OF APPLICATION
COUGH	Blue tansy, chamomile, cypress, fir needle, frankincense, lavender, lemon, pine, rosalina, spearmint, spruce, tea tree	INHALATION, TOPICAL
DEPRESSION	Bergamot, chamomile, clary sage, frankincense, geranium, grapefruit, lavender, neroli, patchouli, petitgrain, sandalwood, sweet orange, ylang-ylang	INHALATION
DIZZINESS	Chamomile, cypress, fir needle, frankincense, ginger, grapefruit, juniper, lavender, lemon, rosalina, spearmint, sweet orange	INHALATION
EAR INFECTION	Chamomile, frankincense, lavender, marjoram, palmarosa, rosalina, tea tree	TOPICAL
EDEMA AND SWELLING	Chamomile, cypress, geranium, ginger, grapefruit, juniper, lavender, lemon, rosalina, spearmint, tea tree	BATH, MASSAGE, TOPICAL
FETAL POSITIONING	Rosalina, spearmint	MASSAGE, TOPICAL
GROUP B STREP/ BACTERIAL VAGINOSIS	Lavender, palmarosa, rosalina, tea tree	BATH, TOPICAL
HEADACHES	Black pepper, blue tansy, chamomile, cypress, fir needle, frankincense, helichrysum, juniper, lavender, marjoram, neroli, petitgrain, rosalina, spearmint	BATH, INHALATION, MASSAGE, TOPICAL
HEARTBURN	Bergamot, chamomile, coriander, cypress, ginger, grapefruit, lavender, lemon, marjoram, neroli, sweet orange, spearmint	INHALATION, TOPICAL
HEMORRHOIDS	Cedarwood, chamomile, cypress, frankincense, geranium, helichrysum, juniper, sandal	BATH, TOPICAL

→

AILMENT	SUGGESTED ESSENTIAL OILS	METHODS OF APPLICATION
INSOMNIA	Bergamot, cedarwood, chamomile, coriander, frankincense, lavender, mandarin, petitgrain, sandalwood, sweet orange, vetiver	BATH, INHALATION, MASSAGE, TOPICAL
LEG CRAMPS	Chamomile, cypress, fir needle, frankincense, helichrysum, juniper, lavender, lemon, marjoram, petitgrain, rosalina	BATH, MASSAGE, TOPICAL
MORNING SICKNESS	Bergamot, chamomile, ginger, grapefruit, lemon, petitgrain, spearmint, sweet orange	INHALATION
PRE-ECLAMPSIA	Bergamot, blue tansy, chamomile, coriander, frankincense, geranium, lavender, mandarin, petitgrain, rosalina, sandalwood, sweet orange, vetiver, ylang-ylang	INHALATION, MASSAGE, ROOM SPRAY, TOPICAL
PREGNANCY FATIGUE	Bergamot, coriander, cypress, fir needle, geranium, ginger, grapefruit, lemon, lemon eucalyptus, pine	INHALATION, MASSAGE, TOPICAL
PUPPP	Blue tansy, chamomile, geranium, helichrysum, lavender, patchouli, rosalina, sandalwood, spearmint	BATH, TOPICAL
ROUND LIGAMENT PAINS	Black pepper, blue tansy, chamomile, cypress, fir needle, frankincense, ginger, helichrysum, lavender, marjoram, petitgrain, rosalina, sandalwood, spearmint, ylang-ylang	MASSAGE, TOPICAL
SCIATICA	Black pepper, cypress, fir needle, lavender, marjoram, petitgrain, rosalina, spearmint, turmeric	BATH, MASSAGE, TOPICAL
STRETCH MARKS	Blue tansy, chamomile, frankincense, geranium, helichrysum, lavender, lemon, neroli, patchouli, sandalwood	MASSAGE, TOPICAL

AILMENT	SUGGESTED ESSENTIAL OILS	METHODS OF APPLICATION
URINARY TRACT INFECTIONS	Lavender, rosalina, tea tree	BATH, TOPICAL
VARICOSE VEINS	Blue tansy, cedarwood, chamomile, cypress, fir needle, frankincense, geranium, ginger, grapefruit, helichrysum, juniper, lavender, lemon, neroli, rosalina, sandalwood	BATH, MASSAGE, TOPICAL
YEAST INFECTIONS	Cedarwood, chamomile, coriander, frankincense, geranium, grapefruit, lavender, lemon, mandarin, sweet orange, tangerine, tea tree	TOPICAL

Labor and Delivery, Postpartum, and Breastfeeding

AILMENT	SUGGESTED ESSENTIAL OILS	METHODS OF APPLICATION
ANXIETY	Bergamot, chamomile, clary sage, coriander, grapefruit, lavender, lemon, neroli, petitgrain, sandalwood, sweet orange, vanilla, ylang-ylang	INHALATION, ROOM SPRAY
AFTER PAINS	Balsam fir, bergamot, black pepper, chamomile, coriander, cypress, fir needle, geranium, ginger, helichrysum, jasmine, lavender, lemon, marjoram, petitgrain, rosalina, spruce, tangerine	COMPRESS, MASSAGE, TOPICAL
BACK LABOR	Bergamot, black pepper, chamomile, coriander, cypress, fir needle, frankincense, ginger, helichrysum, lavender, lemon, marjoram, petitgrain, rosalina, tangerine, spruce	MASSAGE, TOPICAL, LINIMENT
BACK PAINS	Balsam fir, bergamot, black pepper, chamomile, coriander, cypress, fir needle, frankincense, ginger, helichrysum, lavender, lemon, marjoram, petitgrain, rosalina, tangerine, spruce, turmeric	LINIMENT, MASSAGE, TOPICAL

AILMENT	SUGGESTED ESSENTIAL OILS	METHODS OF APPLICATION
BLOCKED DUCTS AND MASTITIS	Balsam fir, bergamot, black pepper, chamomile, coriander, cypress, fir needle, frankincense, ginger, helichrysum, lemon, lavender, marjoram, neroli, rosalina, spruce, tangerine	COMPRESS, MASSAGE, TOPICAL
BLOOD PRESSURE	Bergamot, blue tansy, cedarwood, chamomile, clary sage, coriander, frankincense, lavender, mandarin, marjoram, petitgrain, rosalina, sandalwood, tangerine, vanilla, vetiver, ylang-ylang	INHALATION
CONTRACTIONS	Bergamot, chamomile, cedarwood, coriander, cypress, fir needle, frankincense, grapefruit, juniper, lavender, lemon, lemon eucalyptus, patchouli, petitgrain, rosalina, spearmint, sweet orange	INHALATION, MASSAGE, TOPICAL
C-SECTION CARE	Cedarwood, chamomile, frankincense, geranium, helichrysum, lavender, lemon, neroli, palmarosa, sweet orange, tangerine	INHALATION, TOPICAL, WASH
EPISIOTOMY CARE	Chamomile, cypress, fir needle, frankincense, geranium, helichrysum, lavender, lemon, marjoram, palmarosa, patchouli, sandalwood, sweet orange, tangerine, tea tree	BATH, TOPICAL, WASH
FATIGUE DURING LABOR	Bergamot, black pepper, cedarwood, coriander, fir needle, geranium, ginger, grapefruit, juniper, lemon, palmarosa, petitgrain, pine, spearmint, spruce, sweet orange, tangerine	INHALATION, ROOM SPRAY
GERM KILLING	Bergamot, cedarwood, chamomile, coriander, cypress, fir needle, frankincense, geranium, grapefruit, helichrysum, lavender, lemon, mandarin, marjoram, neroli, petitgrain, rosalina, sandalwood, sweet orange, tangerine	INHALATION, HAND SOAP, TOPICAL

➤

AILMENT	SUGGESTED ESSENTIAL OILS	METHODS OF APPLICATION
HAIR LOSS	Black pepper, cedarwood, chamomile, clary sage, coriander, cypress, fir needle, frankincense, geranium, juniper, lavender, lemon, palmarosa, patchouli, pine, sandalwood, spearmint, sweet orange, tea tree, vetiver, ylang-ylang	MASSAGE, SPRAY, TOPICAL
MILK PRODUCTION	Clary sage, fenugreek, geranium	LINIMENT, MASSAGE, TOPICAL
NAUSEA	Bergamot, chamomile, dill weed, ginger, grapefruit, lemon, mandarin, spearmint, sweet orange, tangerine	INHALATION, TOPICAL
NIPPLES (DRY/CRACKED)	Blue tansy, chamomile, geranium, helichrysum, lavender, neroli, rose, sweet orange	TOPICAL
POSTPARTUM DEPRESSION	Bergamot, cedarwood, chamomile, clary sage, coriander, geranium, grapefruit, lavender, lemon, neroli, petitgrain, sandalwood, sweet orange, vanilla, ylang-ylang	BODY SPRAY, INHALATION, TOPICAL
POSTPARTUM VAGINAL CARE	Cedarwood, chamomile, cypress, fir needle, frankincense, helichrysum, lavender, lemon, mandarin, marjoram, neroli, patchouli, sandalwood, sweet orange, tea tree	BATH, COMPRESS, TOPICAL
SORE BREASTS	Blue tansy, chamomile, frankincense, geranium, ginger, helichrysum, lavender, marjoram, patchouli, petitgrain, rosalina, sandalwood, ylang-ylang	COMPRESS, MASSAGE, TOPICAL
SPEED UP LABOR	Coriander, cypress, fir needle, frankincense, geranium, jasmine, juniper, lavender, rose, ylang-ylang	INHALATION
TRANSITION	Bergamot, chamomile, clary sage, coriander, frankincense, lemon, mandarin, sweet orange, tangerine, vanilla	INHALATION, ROOM SPRAY, TOPICAL

Infants and Young Children

AILMENT	SUGGESTED ESSENTIAL OILS	METHODS OF APPLICATION
ALLERGIES (HAY FEVER)	Blue tansy, chamomile, citronella, cypress, fir needle, frankincense, grapefruit, juniper, lavender, lemon, pine, rosalina, spearmint, spruce, sweet orange	INHALATION
ANXIETY	Bergamot, cedarwood, chamomile, coriander, frankincense, sandalwood, sweet orange, vanilla	INHALATION, MASSAGE, ROOM SPRAY, TOPICAL
ASTHMA	Blue tansy, chamomile, citronella, cypress, fir needle, frankincense, grapefruit, juniper, lavender, lemon, lemon eucalyptus, pine, rosalina, spearmint, spruce, sweet orange	BATH, INHALATION, TOPICAL
ATHLETE'S FOOT	Cedarwood, chamomile, coriander, frankincense, geranium, grapefruit, lavender, lemon, mandarin, pine, tangerine, tea tree	BATH, TOPICAL
BALANITIS	Chamomile, geranium, lavender, palmarosa, tea tree	BATH, TOPICAL
BEDTIME FEARS	Chamomile, lavender, tangerine, vanilla	INHALATION, ROOM SPRAY
BLISTERS	Cedarwood, chamomile, cypress, fir needle, geranium, lavender, lemon, marjoram, neroli, palmarosa, petitgrain, rosalina, lavender, sweet orange, tea tree	BATH, TOPICAL, WASH
BRONCHITIS	Chamomile, cypress, fir needle, frankincense, ginger, lavender, lemon, marjoram, palmarosa, petitgrain, pine, rosalina, sandalwood, spearmint, spruce, tea tree	INHALATION, MASSAGE, SHOWER STEAMERS, TOPICAL
BUG BITES AND STINGS	Blue tansy, chamomile, coriander, cypress, frankincense, geranium, juniper, lavender, marjoram, neroli, palmarosa, patchouli, petitgrain, pine, rosalina, rose, sandalwood, spearmint, tea tree	TOPICAL

➔

AILMENT	SUGGESTED ESSENTIAL OILS	METHODS OF APPLICATION
BUG REPELLENTS	Cedarwood, geranium, grapefruit, lavender, lemon, mandarin, marjoram, patchouli, pine, rosalina, spearmint, sweet orange, tangerine, tea tree	BODY SPRAY, CANDLES, TOPICAL
BURNS AND SUNBURNS	Blue tansy, chamomile, frankincense, geranium, lavender, rosalina, spearmint	TOPICAL
CATARRH	Chamomile, cypress, fir needle, frankincense, ginger, lavender, marjoram, palmarosa, petitgrain, pine, rosalina, sandalwood, spearmint, spruce, tea tree	INHALATION, SALT STEAM, TOPICAL
CHICKEN POX	Coriander, frankincense, geranium, lavender, marjoram, neroli, palmarosa, petitgrain, rose, spearmint, sweet orange, tea tree	BATH, INHALATION, TOPICAL
CIRCUMCISION	Lavender hydrosol	COMPRESS, TOPICAL, WASH
COLDS	Cinnamon, cypress, fir needle, frankincense, lavender, lemon, marjoram, palmarosa, rosalina, spearmint, tea tree	BATH, INHALATION, TOPICAL
COLD SORES	Chamomile, coriander, geranium, lavender, lemon, rosalina, tea tree	TOPICAL
COLIC	Roman chamomile hydrosol	BATH, SPRAY, TOPICAL
CONGESTION	Cedarwood, cypress, fir needle, frankincense, juniper, lavender, lemon, lemon eucalyptus, rosalina, pine, spearmint, spruce, tea tree	INHALATION, SALT STEAM
CONSTIPATION	Chamomile, coriander, dill weed, frankincense, ginger, lemon, petitgrain, spearmint, sweet orange	MASSAGE, TOPICAL

➤

AILMENT	SUGGESTED ESSENTIAL OILS	METHODS OF APPLICATION
COUGH	Chamomile, cypress, fir needle, frankincense, ginger, lavender, marjoram, petitgrain, pine, rosalina, sandalwood, spearmint, spruce	INHALATION, MASSAGE, TOPICAL
CRADLE CAP	Lavender hydrosol	TOPICAL
CROUP	Black pepper, cedarwood, chamomile, cypress, frankincense, lavender, lemon, marjoram, palmarosa, pine, rosalina, sandalwood, spruce	INHALATION, MASSAGE, TOPICAL
CUTS AND SCRAPES	Blue tansy, cedarwood, chamomile, cypress, fir needle, frankincense, geranium, helichrysum, lavender, lemon, palmarosa, rose, sweet orange, tea tree	TOPICAL, WASH
DANDRUFF	Bergamot, cedarwood, chamomile, cinnamon, coriander, fir needle, geranium, grapefruit, lavender, lemon, palmarosa, patchouli, petitgrain, rosalina, sandalwood, sweet orange, tangerine, tea tree	SPRAY, TOPICAL
DIAPER RASH	Blue tansy, chamomile, frankincense, geranium, lavender, lemon, neroli, palmarosa, petitgrain, rosalina, sweet orange	TOPICAL, WASH
DIARRHEA	Chamomile, dill weed, ginger, lavender, lemon, petitgrain, spearmint, sweet orange	MASSAGE, TOPICAL
DRY SKIN	Blue tansy, carrot seed, cedarwood, chamomile, coriander, frankincense, geranium, grapefruit, helichrysum, lavender, lemon, palmarosa, patchouli, petitgrain, rosalina, rose, sandalwood, sweet orange	TOPICAL
EARACHES AND EAR INFECTIONS	Chamomile, frankincense, lavender, marjoram, palmarosa, rosalina, tea tree	MASSAGE, TOPICAL

➜

AILMENT	SUGGESTED ESSENTIAL OILS	METHODS OF APPLICATION
ECZEMA AND PSORIASIS	Blue tansy, cedarwood, chamomile, coriander, frankincense, geranium, helichrysum, lavender, neroli, palmarosa, patchouli, tea tree	TOPICAL, WASH
FEVER	Chamomile, coriander, cypress, fir needle, grapefruit, lavender, lemon, marjoram, neroli, palmarosa, petitgrain, rosalina, spearmint, tea tree	BATH, COMPRESS
GERM KILLING AND IMMUNE BOOSTING	Bergamot, cedarwood, chamomile, coriander, cypress, frankincense, geranium, grapefruit, helichrysum, lavender, lemon, mandarin, marjoram, neroli, petitgrain, rosalina, sandalwood, sweet orange, tangerine, tea tree	INHALATION, TOPICAL
GROWING PAINS	Chamomile, coriander, cypress, fir needle, helichrysum, juniper, lavender, lemon, marjoram, rosalina, turmeric	BATH, MASSAGE, TOPICAL
HAND, FOOT, AND MOUTH DISEASE	Chamomile, coriander, geranium, helichrysum, lavender, neroli, palmarosa, petitgrain, rosalina, sandalwood, sweet orange, tea tree	TOPICAL, WASH
HEADACHES	Black pepper, blue tansy, chamomile, cypress, fir needle, frankincense, ginger, helichrysum, juniper, lavender, marjoram, neroli, petitgrain, rosalina, spearmint	INHALATION, TOPICAL
HEAD LICE	Cedarwood, geranium, lavender, palmarosa, patchouli, rosalina, spearmint, sweet orange, tea tree	TOPICAL
HEAT RASH AND HEAT EXHAUSTION	Bergamot, blue tansy, chamomile, clary sage, cypress, fir needle, juniper, lemon, palmarosa, rosalina, spearmint	BATH, COMPRESS, SPRAY
HIVES	Blue tansy, chamomile, helichrysum, lavender, lemon, neroli, palmarosa, rosalina, tea tree	COMPRESS, TOPICAL

➜

AILMENT	SUGGESTED ESSENTIAL OILS	METHODS OF APPLICATION
INFLUENZA	Bergamot, blue tansy, chamomile, cinnamon leaf, coriander, cypress, fir needle, grapefruit, juniper, lavender, lemon, marjoram, palmarosa, petitgrain, rosalina, sweet orange, tangerine, tea tree	INHALATION, TOPICAL
NAUSEA AND VOMITING	Bergamot, chamomile, dill weed, ginger, grapefruit, lemon, mandarin, spearmint, sweet orange, tangerine	INHALATION
PNEUMONIA	Cedarwood, coriander, chamomile, cypress, fir needle, frankincense, ginger, juniper, lavender, lemon, lemon eucalyptus, marjoram, palmarosa, petitgrain, rosalina, spearmint, sweet orange, tea tree	INHALATION, SHOWER STEAMERS, TOPICAL
POISON IVY, OAK, AND SUMAC	Blue tansy, chamomile, cypress, fir needle, frankincense, geranium, juniper, neroli, pine, lavender, marjoram, neroli, palmarosa, patchouli, rosalina, rose, sandalwood, spearmint, tea tree	BATH, TOPICAL
RINGWORM	Cedarwood, chamomile, coriander, frankincense, geranium, grapefruit, lavender, mandarin, rosalina, sweet orange, tangerine, tea tree	TOPICAL
SLEEP	Bergamot, cedarwood, chamomile, clary sage, coriander, frankincense, lavender, lemon, mandarin, marjoram, neroli, petitgrain, rosalina, sandalwood, sweet orange, tangerine, valerian root, vanilla, ylang-ylang	BATH, INHALATION, MASSAGE, TOPICAL
SNEEZING	Blue tansy, chamomile, cypress, fir needle, geranium, juniper, lavender, lemon, rosalina, rose, spearmint	INHALATION
SNIFFLES AND RUNNY NOSE	Blue tansy, cedarwood, chamomile, cypress, fir needle, juniper, lavender, lemon, marjoram, palmarosa, rosalina, spearmint, spruce, tea tree	INHALATION

AILMENT	SUGGESTED ESSENTIAL OILS	METHODS OF APPLICATION
SORE THROAT	Chamomile, frankincense, geranium, ginger, helichrysum, lavender, lemon, marjoram, rosalina, spearmint, tea tree	SPRAY, TOPICAL
TEETHING	Chamomile, lavender	TOPICAL
THRUSH	Blue tansy, chamomile, frankincense, geranium, helichrysum, lavender, lemon, neroli, palmarosa, petitgrain, rosalina, spearmint, sweet orange, tea tree	TOPICAL
UMBILICAL CORD INFECTIONS	Lavender hydrosol	TOPICAL
WARTS	Cedarwood, cypress, geranium, lavender, lemon, marjoram, rosalina, tea tree	TOPICAL

Trusted Essential Oil Brands

AURA CACIA

One of the most widely recognized brands in local retail shops and grocery store, Aura Cacia has been selling quality essential oils since 1982. They source all of their ingredients carefully and sustainably, and test every shipment of essential oils they receive to verify their purity and quality.

WHERE TO BUY   You can purchase Aura Cacia essential oils in many local and national natural foods stores as well as on their website (AuraCacia.com), on Amazon, and on other Internet grocery stores.

RATING   4/5 stars

TOP FEATURES   They source their ingredients sustainably, they support several organizations that help women transform their lives, and their essential oil blends smell great.

EDENS GARDEN

Born from the idea that an essential oil company should care more about the people using their essential oils than they do about the bottom line, one mother created Edens Garden essential oils from the ground up. Edens Garden is a family-owned company that sells quality pure essential oils direct, without the middleman.

WHERE TO BUY   Edens Garden oils can be found both on their website (EdensGarden.com) and on Amazon. If you are purchasing through Amazon, be sure you are buying from their official storefront and not an unknown seller, to prevent any possible adulteration.

RATING   4/5 stars

TOP FEATURES   They sell an entire line of essential oil safe blends made specifically for children, they have great prices, and they source their essential oils from quality sources.

MOUNTAIN ROSE HERBS

This herb and essential oil company based in Oregon strives to sell high-quality, organic herbs, essential oils, beauty clays, and other natural ingredients, while also living by their strict green and eco-friendly standards. They're certified organic by Oregon Tilth and the USDA, Earth Kosher-certified, Fair Trade-certified, and most impressively, a certified zero-waste company.

WHERE TO BUY   You can find their herbs, essential oils, and ingredients on their website (MountainRoseHerbs.com).

RATING   5/5 stars

TOP FEATURES   All their essential oils are certified organic, they are the most eco-friendly option, their pricing is fantastic, you can purchase all of the organic herbs and ingredients you might need to make your own health and beauty products, too, they support several nonprofit organizations, including ones that help watershed conservation and endangered plant conservation.

NOW FOODS

Now Foods has been in the natural food and supplement industry since 1948. They are well known in the health food industry as a company that sells a wide variety of high-quality health products at affordable prices.

WHERE TO BUY   You can purchase Now Foods essential oils in many local natural foods grocery stores as well as online (NowFoods.com); on Amazon, and on other Internet grocery stores.

RATING   3/5 stars

TOP FEATURES   Their products can be found everywhere, are affordable, and they have a variety of single oils and blends to choose from.

PLANT THERAPY

Plant Therapy is an essential oil company that is looking to positively impact as many lives as "humanly possible." They feel that providing customers with excellent service and high-quality products at affordable prices will help them impact the world. On a mission to educate the world on safe essential oil use, Plant Therapy teamed up with aromatherapy safety expert Robert Tisserand to create the first line of kid-safe essential oil blends and singles. They also worked closely with Tisserand to organoleptically test their oils before sending them off to a third-party testing facility. Plant Therapy is a business based on family values and caring for the people that keep them going.

WHERE TO BUY   You can find Plant Therapy essential oils on their website (PlantTherapy.com) and on Amazon.

RATING   5/5 stars

TOP FEATURES   Kid-safe essential oils designed by Robert Tisserand, they are affordable, their customer service is impeccable, the shipping prices are modest, they test every essential oil batch that comes through their doors and won't sell it if it doesn't meet their strict quality standards, and, most importantly, they have a team of certified aromatherapists on hand to answer your essential oil safety questions.

Mini Glossary

ABORTIFACIENT Capable of inducing a miscarriage

ANALGESIC Pain relieving

ANTIBACTERIAL Fights the growth of bacteria

ANTIDEPRESSANT Helps counteract depression and lifts the mood

ANTIFUNGAL Prevents the growth of fungi

ANTISEPTIC Prevents the growth of bacteria

CARRIER OIL A fatty, neutral oil (such as avocado seed oil, coconut oil, grapeseed oil, or olive oil) used to dilute essential oils

CARMINATIVE Helps relieve flatulence, ease gripping pains, and settles the digestive system

EXPECTORANT Helps get rid of catarrh, phlegm, and mucus

HYDROSOL These gentle herbal-infused waters are made from the condensate of water distilled with plant material. The resulting waters are completely infused with the essence of the plant, with the essential oils sitting on the top of the hydrosol. After gently removing the essential oils for bottling, a little bit of essential oil remains emulsified in the waters. These plant waters contain all of the same healing components of the herbs and can be used in place of water in many natural beauty and cosmetics recipes.

NEAT Using an essential oil undiluted, without a carrier oil

VOLATILE A substance, like an essential oil, that is unstable and evaporates quickly

References

Buckle, Jane. *Clinical Aromatherapy: Essential Oils in Healthcare.* 3rd ed. St. Louis, MO: Churchill Livingstone, 2014.

Burt, S.A., and R.D. Reinders. "Antibacterial Activity of Selected Plant Essential Oils against Escherichia coli O157:H7." *Letters in Applied Microbiology* 36, no. 3 (2003):162-7. www.ncbi.nlm.nih.gov/pubmed/12581376.

Centers for Disease Control and Prevention. "Ear Infection." *Get Smart: Know When Antibiotics Work in Doctors' Offices.* Last modified January 27, 2017. www.cdc.gov/getsmart/community/for-patients/common-illnesses/ear-infection.html.

Clark, Demetria. *Aromatherapy and Herbal Remedies for Pregnancy, Birth, and Breastfeeding.* Summertown, TN: Healthy Living Publications, 2015.

Clarke, Marge. *Essential Oils and Aromatics.* Amazon Digital Services, 2013.

Docteur Valnet Aromathérapie. "Docteur Valnet: Founder of Modern Aromatherapy." Accessed June 23, 2017. www.docteurvalnet.com/fr/content/6-docteur-valnet.

Environmental Working Group. "Greener School Cleaning Supplies: School Cleaner Test Results." November 3, 2009. www.ewg.org/research/greener-school-cleaning-supplies/school-cleaner-test-results?schoolprod=219.

Fox, Kate. "The Smell Report." Social Issues Research Center. Accessed June 23, 2017. www.sirc.org/publik/smell.pdf.

Gattefossé, René-Maurice. *Gattefossé's Aromatherapy.* 2nd revised ed. Ebury Digital, 2012.

Gatti, G., and R. Cayola. "The Action of Essences on the Nervous System." *Rivista Italiana delle Essenze e Profumi* 5, no.12 (1923): 133.

Grumezescu, Alexandru. *Nutraceuticals.* Cambridge, MA: Academic Press, 2016.

Herbal Academy. "Oats Benefits: Getting to Know Avena Sativa." May 12, 2014. www.theherbalacademy.com/oats-benefits-getting-to-know-avena-sativa.

Inouye, S., T. Takizawa, and H. Yamaguchi. "Antibacterial Activity of Essential Oils and Their Major Constituents Against Respiratory Tract Pathogens by Gaseous Contact." *Journal of Antimicrobial Chemotherapy* 47, no. 5 (May 2001): 565-573. www.academic.oup.com/jac/article/47/5/565/858508/Antibacterial-activity-of-essential-oils-and-their.

Lawless, Julia. *The Encyclopedia of Essential Oils: The Complete Guide to the Use of Aromatic Oils in Aromatherapy, Herbalism, Health & Well-Being.* Newburyport, MA: Conari Press, 2013.

Lillehei A.S., and L.L. Halcon. "A Systematic Review of the Effect of Inhaled Essential Oils on Sleep." *Journal of Alternative and Complementary Medicine* 20, no. 6 (June 2014): 441-451. www.ncbi.nlm.nih.gov/pubmed/24720812.

National Institute for Occupational Safety and Health. "Reproductive Health and the Workplace." April 20, 2017. www.cdc.gov/niosh/topics/repro/solvents.html.

Oils and Plants. "Jean Valnet." Accessed June 23, 2017. www.oilsandplants.com/valnet.htm.

Prabuseenivasan, S., M. Jayakumar, and S. Ignacimuthu. "In Vitro Antibacterial Activity of Some Plant Essential Oils." *BMC Complement Alternative Medicine* 6, no. 39 (November 2006): 196-207. www.ncbi.nlm.nih.gov/pmc/articles/PMC1693916

Price, Shirley. *Aromatherapy Workbook: A Complete Guide to Understanding and Using Essential Oils*. London, UK: Thorsons, 2012. Kindle edition.

Raho, B., and M. Benali. "Antibacterial Activity of the Essential Oils from the Leaves of Eucalyptus globulus against Escherichia coli and Staphylococcus aureus." *Asian Pacific Journal of Tropical Biomedicine* 2, no. 9 (Septempter 2012): 739-742. www.ncbi.nlm.nih.gov/pmc/articles/PMC3609378/

Silva, G., C. Luft, A. Lunardelli, et al. "Antioxidant, Analgesic and Anti-inflammatory Effects of Lavender Essential Oil." *Anais da Academia Brasileira de Ciências* 87, no. 2 (August 2015): 1397-408. www.ncbi.nlm.nih.gov/pubmed/26247152

Smith, Anne. "Drugs and Breastfeeding." *Breastfeeding Basics*. Last modified September 2015. Accessed June 23, 2017. www.breastfeedingbasics.com/articles/drugs-and-breastfeeding.

Stea, Susanna, Alina Beraudi, and Dalila De Pasquale. "Essential Oils for Complementary Treatment of Surgical Patients: State of the Art." *Evidence-Based Complementary Alternatative Medicine* (2014): 726341. www.ncbi.nlm.nih.gov/pmc/articles/PMC3953654.

Tisserand, Robert. "Gattefossé's Burn." April 22, 2001. www.roberttisserand.com/2011/04/gattefosses-burn.

Tisserand, Robert, and Rodney Young. *Essential Oil Safety*. 2nd ed. St. Louis, MO: Churchill Livingstone, 2013.

Webb, Becky. "How To Turn a Breech Baby Naturally." *Rooted Blessings*. June 26, 2014. www.rootedblessings.com/how-to-turn-a-breech-baby-naturally

Weir, Kirsten. "Scents and Sensibility." *American Psychological Association* 42, no. 2 (February 2011): 40. www.apa.org/monitor/2011/02/scents.aspx.

Worwood, Valerie Ann. *Aromatherapy for the Healthy Child*. Novato, CA: New World Library, 2012.

Yavari Kia, P., et al. "The Effect of Lemon Inhalation Aromatherapy on Nausea and Vomiting of Pregnancy: A Double-Blinded, Randomized, Controlled Clinical Trial." *Iranian Red Crescent Medical Journal* 16, no. 3 (March 2014):e14360. doi: 10.5812/ircmj.14360.

Index of Remedies by Essential Oil

Index

science of, 7–8

tools and equipment, 32–33

trusted brands, 259–260

Essential Oil Safety, 23

Essential Oils and Aromatics, 12

F

Fatigue

labor and delivery, 94–95, 251

pregnancy, 68–69, 249

Fennel, 20–21

Fenugreek, 20

Fetal positioning, 55–56, 248

Fever blisters. *See* Cold sores

Fevers, 175–176, 256. *See also* Cold and flu

First aid

blisters, 125–128, 253

bug bites and stings, 131–133, 253

burns and sunburns, 136–138, 254

cuts and scrapes, 159–161, 255

dry/cracked nipples, 101–102, 252

Fixed oils. *See* Carrier oils

Flu. *See* Cold and flu

Fungal infections

athlete's foot, 119–121, 253

balanitis, 122–123, 253

dandruff, 162–163, 255

diaper rash, 164–166, 255

dry skin, 169–170, 255

ringworm, 198–200, 257

thrush, 209–211

yeast infections, 79, 250

G

Galactagogues, 98

Gattefossé, René-Maurice, 4

Gatti, Giovanni, 6

Germ killing. *See also* Bacterial infections; Fungal infections; Viral infections

infants and young children, 177–178, 256

postpartum, 96–97, 251

Ginger, 15

Goat's rue, 21

Grapeseed oil, 14

Group B strep, 56–57, 248

Growing pains, 178–180, 256

H

Hair loss, 97–98, 252

Hand, foot, and mouth disease, 180–181, 256

Hay fever. *See* Allergies

Headaches

infants and young children, 182–183, 256

pregnancy, 58–59, 248

Head lice, 183–185, 256

Heartburn, 59–60, 248

Heat rash and heat exhaustion, 186–188, 256

Hemorrhoids, 61–62, 248

Hemp seed oil, 14

Herbs

anti-inflammatory, 106, 107, 120, 127, 149, 161, 179, 180, 189

lactation promoting, 20–21

pregnancy supporting, 15

Herpes simplex1 virus (HSV-1), 147

Hives, 189–190, 256

Honey, 156

Hydrosols, 12

I

Immune boosting, 177–178, 256

Infants and young children. *See also specific ailments*

oils that are safe for, 27–29

safety guidelines, 19, 22–23

About the Author

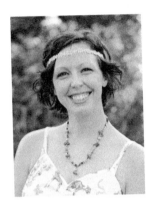

CHRISTINA ANTHIS is the hippy behind the blog TheHippyHomemaker.com. After years of surgeries, pain, poor health, and narcolepsy, Christina realized that her poor diet and the toxic chemicals in her life were making her family sick. Fed up, she decided to take her family's health into her own hands and began training in aromatherapy and herbalism. As she learned how to change her own life, she began sharing her journey on her blog, helping others to live healthier, hippier lives themselves. Christina writes about green and eco-friendly living, aromatherapy, herbalism, holistic health, and natural beauty.

CPSIA information can be obtained
at www.ICGtesting.com
Printed in the USA
BVOW10s0952250717
490164BV00005B/6/P